Roots

A Chronicle of Peace

Julius M. Sweet

Table of Contents

Dedication

Dedicated to God who led the way, to my wife, who supported and inspired me to succeed, and to the loved ones who helped shape this story and make the author into the person he is today.

Acknowledgements

So that it may be known that the families, loved ones, and friends in this story have all been forgiven and prayed for. This story is not meant to shed blame or accuse anyone. The purpose of it is to tell a truthful and honest story based on Warren Peace, a third-person character created to relive the author's personal story and the historical events it parallels. With sincere hope, this story serves as a light and a guide in its reader's life and in their darkest times. I pray the lessons learned, the path to forgiveness and the personal freedom Warren experiences in this story will empower you to heal, assume your role in society, and take control of your life.

About the Author

The author of this book and founder of The Sweet Ethics Residential Association (SERA), Julius M. Sweet, saw the impact of mental illness and substance abuse on his family, loved ones, and community. This book chronicles the upbringing and story of the author and does so from the third-person perspective. The author hopes this story can help and guide those who have lived or who are currently living similar scenarios. Readers will follow Warren Peace through his family history, childhood, adolescence and adulthood as he overcomes obstacles, endures many challenges, and seeks to rise above his own inner demons to create something greater than himself and that can, in turn, help the world.

You can visit the author's nonprofit organization here: www.sweetethicsra.org

Chapter I: Summer

Summer Lopez was born on the Northern island Luzon in the Philippines shortly after the start of the Korean War and between World War II and the Vietnam War. Not much is known of her early childhood life other than her ancestry which, although mostly Filipino, also descends from China, Southern India, and Basque. Sometime during the Vietnam War, between 1965-75, Summer met a US sailor on Luzon, near Manila. She married him and gave birth to a son and daughter in Olongapo in the Subic Bay Area. Soon after, her family disowned her as they saw her marriage to an American dishonorable. Summer's new military family then rotated to the USA, where they gave birth to a third child in Chicago, Illinois. One day after work, Summer's husband came home and found their three children home alone. There was no note and Summer was gone. This family would never see her again.

When Dominic Peace met Summer in Stockton, California, almost 10 years later, in the year 1989, she had two children with her, a girl and a boy. Dominic's family had moved up from Phoenix, Arizona, about nine years prior after a long, tragic history there. He and Summer quickly became acquainted, and soon, they were in a relationship with one another and gave birth to a son, her last child and Dominic's only child, and they named him Warren Peace.

Dominic descends from a family with blood roots in the American South: Louisiana, East Texas, and Arkansas. His father's bloodline also descended from the early African Americans of Virginia. Dominic's mother, Stella Peace, who would eventually become Warren's guardian, was born in Florence, Arizona. Stella's mother, Madea, was born near Dallas, Texas, in a small town named Corsicana in 1923. Madea was a product of rape. Her mother had been employed to clean the house of a white man of Anglo Saxon and Scandinavian descent, while her husband was away preoccupied with military duty. The head of the household forced himself on her; nine months later, she conceived Madea. Still, Madea was accepted by her mother's husband when he returned from duty and he gave her his family surname, Nunn. Madea had a rough childhood and upbringing. According to those who told Warren, Madea grew up during a time when it was not okay to be black and white. Madea, although black, was very light complexed. When Warren visited her in 1997 with his grandmother and cousins while she lay in a Las Vegas nursing home because of a stroke that paralyzed her, he didn't see a hint of brown in her.

Madea married three times in her life and gave birth to several children. The second of which was Stella, Warren's Grandmother, whose father was black and Cherokee. When Stella turned twelve years old, she voluntarily attended

2

church and worshipped God like none other. She was of the Church of God in Christ (COGIC) faith. While in church one day in Arizona, she met a man named Samuel Peace and they fell in love. Samuel and his large family, although black, also descend from the Cherokee. Soon, Samuel and Stella gave birth to three children, the second of which was Dominic. Dominic didn't remember Samuel very well. To him, his father was nonexistent in his life until he had to attend his funeral when he was 14 years old. Samuel had left the family shortly after the birth of his children and illegally married another woman named Odessa. She bore him two sons before discovering he was still married to Stella. Samuel shortly afterward moved to Houston, Texas, in the mid-70's. He moved in with his eldest sibling, Lee Ethyl Peace and her husband and took a job as a warehouse worker for a toy company. On April 1st, 1977, around 2 AM, Samuel was shot and killed by his 26-year-old white coworker, a French Canadian named James Paul Michaud, who had laid in to wait for him in the warehouse entryway after work. What got discovered was Samuel had manufactured a toy that was about to get him promoted and James started to steal from him. When the issue got reported to management, James retaliated by shooting him thirteen times with two pistols. In the police report Warren requested years later, he read that his grandfather's killer had been drinking whiskey and the half-empty bottle was found in between his dead body and the front door to the warehouse. Samuel's body was flown back to Arizona to be buried beside his parents in Yuma and his killer would spend less than forty days in jail before he got deported. Although separated, Samuel's life insurance got awarded to Stella after it had been found the pair were still legally married despite Stella's attempt to serve him divorce papers which he did not sign. Stella had been remarried, bore other children, and was now a single mother and a matriarch. She reverted her last name back to her first husband's surname – 'Peace'.

Warren believes his dad's problems started at a very young age when Dominic was around the age of four. Just after Dominic's father left, Stella gave birth to a fourth child, a baby girl named Justina. Dominic told Warren the story of when he and his older brother, Curt, had to babysit Justina, who was sick with pneumonia, because their mother was going to church. While Stella was at church in another neighborhood, a black teenage girl knocked on the door and told Dominic and his older brother that their mother requested they give Justina to her. The two brothers handed their baby sister over to the girl and never saw either of them again. There was a church across the street from the house, and the girl carried Justina to it, wrapped a diaper around her neck, and hung her from a knob on its front door. Warren would later see the newspaper clipping from this tragedy in one of his grandmother's albums. The article said the teenage girl had mental health issues, and the baby had died from pneumonia, not from hanging on a church door. A version of this story told by another relative of Warren's named the girl as a babysitter to Justina who hung her in the basement of the church with the help of another girl. After years of tragedy and misfortune in Arizona, Grandma Peace moved the entire family to Stockton, California, around the year 1980. When Dominic and Summer gave birth to Warren in 1990, they moved in with Grandma Peace briefly before getting a place of their own. It wasn't long before that Dominic began to steal full-time. He enjoyed it and saw it as the only means to provide support for himself and his family. Dominic was also good at basketball and could've gone pro. Warren heard one story from his uncles growing up was of a bet Dominic accepted, which was to jump over a Volkswagen beetle and dunk. Dominic soared over the beetle and slammed the ball through to everyone's amazement. Still, he couldn't stay off the streets. Warren accepted the fact his dad, in his earlier years, would rather break into a stranger's house and steal their bike instead of seeking to improve his life and contribute to his community and economy in a positive and appropriate manner.

As Warren was told, Dominic kept on about it until one evening, while riding away on a new bike he had just stolen from a house. A voice and a feeling from within told him to take the bike back. He followed his subconscious and took the bike back to where the police were closing in. They arrested him and then Summer left him and took her children away. When Dominic got out of jail a few months later, he struggled to find Summer and Warren. Summer had relocated her family to downtown Stockton, bought a Ford Pinto, and moved on from Dominic. The day Dominic found them at their apartment is the day Warren can recall as his earliest and first memory. Dominic had approached Warren to take him, but Summer fought him off until the police came. Warren saw the police haul his dad out of the room while Summer hit and screamed at him. Warren never forgot that scene and wouldn't see Dominic again until around nineteen.

A man soon took an interest in Summer, who was a Hispanic named Paul. Warren remembers the day he first met Paul when he was about the age of five. Summer was pushing him in a stroller and they stopped outside the bar where he worked. Warren remembered looking up at the person whom he had no clue was the devil about to be invited to his home. It wasn't long before Paul began to beat Summer. He'd drink, do drugs, and find any reason to attack her. Warren witnessed his mother get struck, choked, and threatened with weapons. One evening, Warren blocked his mother as Paul pulled a crossbow and aimed it at her in the hallway of their downtown apartment building. Warren then pushed, kicked, and screamed at Paul's legs until he put the weapon away. When Warren woke up the next day, he saw Paul had, later into the previous evening, struck Summer with a beer bottle instead, giving her a knot on her forehead and a black eye.

Another evening, Summer left a babysitter with Warren and went out for the night. About 20 minutes after Summer left, the babysitter walked Warren to a house party down the street to buy drugs from a man who sat on the steps of the property. The man, for unknown reasons, lunged from the steps and attacked the babysitter right in front of Warren. He didn't understand why he attacked her, but he figured it had something to do with the transaction. She was badly beaten, bloody, and sobbing. The babysitter walked Warren back to Summer, who was waiting for their return. Summer scolded the babysitter for taking Warren away from the apartment and refused any empathy for her. Sometime after this incident, Summer moved the family to an apartment multiplex near the Delta River and Paul followed. It was here Warren laid flat on his back in the living room, as if on a cross, in front of his family. It was at this moment he felt he wanted to be like the man he had just heard about on the television; a man named Jesus Christ. His brother and sister laughed and ridiculed him and Summer found it intriguing. Summer and Paul's cycle of fighting and drug abuse continued until Thanksgiving Day in 1996 when she was home alone preparing dinner. In a coroner's report Warren read later in his young adult years, Summer reported to a friend by phone she was having chest pains and didn't feel well. Summer went into the restroom while preparing steak for dinner and died instantly from an aneurysm. Warren's sister found Summer when she got home and it changed her life. When Warren got home, there was a gathering of close family friends outside his house. They told Warren that they had taken his mother to the hospital. After waiting in the lobby for what felt like hours and hours on end, Warren was ushered to an upper floor and was crammed into a small office with friends of the family and his sobbing sister. She snapped at Warren before he could laugh at her crying, something apparently, he and his brother used to do, telling him, "You better not laugh, Warren!" However, Warren wasn't sure why she was crying and why everyone had blank looks on their faces. Finally, a nurse stepped in and whispered to one of the adults, "They just wheeled her by." Then the nurse stepped out and the adult communicated Summer had passed away.

Warren had a dream about her that night. In it, she came to visit him as he and his two siblings slept in the living room. He heard his siblings greet her, but he was terrified to look up because she looked as if she had just climbed out of a grave. Warren didn't realize it then, but years later, he figured she was trying to say goodbye.

Chapter II: Grandmother Peace

Warren stayed at his sister's grandmother's house for about a week until his own grandmother, Stella Peace, could come up from Fresno to retrieve him at the request of an incarcerated Dominic. She lived in Stockton a short while after her first arrival to the state, then she moved to Vallejo, and then settled permanently in Fresno. Before Summer's funeral, Warren was split from his sister and brother and taken to Fresno, where the courts granted his grandmother as a legal guardianship. The spirit of the drive down from Stockton was cold and dreary. Warren was worried and filled with uncertainty. He didn't remember his grandma Peace much from before, only that she visited him and his mother when they lived downtown, but he quickly knew her to be strong-handed and short-tempered. He didn't know it then, but the same strict, southern Christian and abusive upbringing that plagued and haunted his dad and his eight other siblings would soon become Warren's own birthright.

Grandma Peace, a matriarch, had reared ten children, including Justina. Warren came to know and refers to her as a 'mother'. Within two weeks, she had accustomed herself to giving him whippings, snapping and yelling, staring him down with cold glares, and putting him on room restriction punishments that can last up to a month with no television or extracurricular privileges. The first hit he took from his grandmother was in the backseat of her brown '88 Ford Taurus. He unintentionally kept kicking the back of her seat as he tried to see out of the window at the City of Fresno. She warned him not to do it again each time he kicked it, or he would get it. Surely enough, he kicked again, and she reached back quick and struck him in the leg with her thick, meaty palm. Although he was taken aback at the action, he knew a blow was coming sooner or later as Grandma Peace had quickly introduced him to her dominating personality upon arrival by threatening him with butt whippings for offenses he didn't even know he committed. Kicking the back of his grandmother's seat and getting a hit for it reminded him of a time when he had to walk with Summer after she enrolled him into preschool near Pacific Ave. They were walking across the street to go back home and Summer stepped onto the curb. Warren tripped her because he thought it would be funny. Summer badly scraped her knee, yelled at him, and didn't talk to him the rest of his way back home. He wasn't struck for the offense although he could tell, even at that age, he had humiliated and hurt his mother. Summer hadn't been dead and buried for a month before Warren started to get beat by his new mother. Grandma Peace reigned entirely over his childhood. Everything and anything Warren did upset his grandmother, and he would seldom take a beating for the offenses he made. The rate and the frequency of the beating would rapidly increase as the years dragged by.

For five years after Summer's death, Warren was made to attend church at Ebenezer COGIC every Sunday and bible study during the week. One day, his grandmother made him kneel in front of the church and told him to pray to Christ. He was on his knees praying, "Thank you, Jesus," for so long that he fell asleep in front of everyone. When he had awakened, after what felt like thirty minutes of napping, his grandma Peace was smiling at him from her first-row bench seat with his cousins sitting still and quietly beside her. This wasn't the only time he had seen her smile. Another day, when they lived in Maple Square apartments (now called Maple Grove) in South Fresno beside Balderas elementary school, where Warren had attended, his grandmother asked him to go to the refrigerator to check for leftovers. He checked and must have missed the Tupperware it was in because he reported to her there wasn't any and went to the laundromat on the apartment complex grounds to attend one of his many assigned chores. As he was checking the clothes, his Aunt Tania entered looking spooked. At this age in his life, this was Warren's favorite aunt. She was also the youngest of Grandma Peace's children. She told him Grandma Peace found leftovers despite what he told her and she had labeled and named him a liar. A liar in the Peace household was a true sinner who was forbidden from anything fun and must be condemned to avoid doing it again.

Aunt Tania encouraged Warren to wait it out and not go back. Warren knew that would only make matters worse. He knew his grandmother's temper and persistence and they wouldn't die down quickly enough. He manned up and went to the apartment and begrudgingly entered his grandmother's bedroom. She was there on the edge of her bed, bouncing up and down, smiling with her legs swinging happily back and forth. She commanded Warren to go to the storage closet on the balcony and pick between a board and an extension cord for his chastisement. He reluctantly chose the board, which used to support one of their beds on its frame, and she beat him with it until his butt turned hot and numb. Warren preferred the board most of the time because belts, belts with rivets, and of course, the extension cord would cut into his skin, create welts and thick bruises, and cause blood to drip down his thighs and legs.

Even in situations in which Warren was not at fault, but his cousins were, he would find himself getting blamed and taking the punishment. Warren was to lead by example, do as told and not as he sees, and adhere to the law of fear and obedience. In any such case of a whooping or beating that Grandma Peace didn't have the energy to muster, she would defer to her son, Victor. On days where she was too weary, she'd load Warren and any other offenders into her Ford Taurus and then drive them up Blackstone Avenue to Uncle Victor's apartment in Fig Garden. Despite this nightmare version, Warren liked Fig Garden in that it was very green and massive. They would also get to drive down Christmas tree lane in the same community every year and he thought it was the most beautiful display of lights and decorations he had ever seen.

One year, Warren trick-or-treated in this community, much to his dread because he had to first meet his cousins at his Uncle Victor's home where they lived. Uncle Victor was scary. He was over six feet tall, big and broadly built, and always had a shaved head. When he walked about, he donned a flared nose, a signature indicator of his incessant bad mood and quick temperedness. This man terrified Warren the most of any other he had met in his young and adult life and he honestly felt his uncle enjoyed it. One day, Warren hadn't done anything wrong in an incident during which his cousins were the culprits and made the trip to Uncle Victor's apartment in Fig Garden anyway. When his uncle came down to collect his soon-to-be victims, Grandma Peace communicated to him that Warren wasn't to get out. However, Uncle Victor ignored her, yelled and threatened Warren, and made him get out of the car. He beat Warren despite the many attempts by his grandmother to stop Victor. Warren had never seen his grandma Peace act so guilty and sad about a whooping imposed on him before, but for this one beating, he felt her sincere apology, although she didn't clearly state one. For the next couple of weeks or so, Warren got a respite from his grandmother's short-tempered and abusive ways. For the first time since living with her, he experienced her kindness. She would buy him something extra when at the store, something she rarely, if ever, did, and most important to Warren was that she would talk to him sweetly. She would do so when she asked or told him anything with a harmonious tone and warm expression. For those couple of weeks, Warren felt as if his grandmother loved him, and still, he knew it was a matter of time before her switch would flip again and she'd become her true self. Sure enough, whatever past pain and turmoil that plagued his grandmother would surely seep back in and remain firm in her being once again, thus unsettling her spirit. Her cycle of abuse with Warren resumed and would continue for five more years.

While in the third grade at Balderas Elementary school, Warren took a reading test and was told he could read at the 11th grade level. This made his grandmother proud and she even told his family. However, for a class party in which Warren had no money to bring anything, he instead decided to steal used items from around his grandmother's apartment, such as hair berets, toys, and clothing items. He loaded everything into a black garbage bag and divided its contents amongst his classmates at the party. The students went on a short break from the party, and when they returned, Warren's teacher told him that she had called his guardian about the gifts and that he would have to return them all to her. Warren dreaded the walk home when school ended and tried to take a long way, but the apartment complex was next door to campus. When he arrived at his grandmother's apartment, he got berated for what he had done and even faced scrutiny from some of his cousins for stealing from them too. However, although he was threatened with a beating, he did not get one.

Warren reasoned that it had a lot to do with his dad, Dominic, and how he used to steal from her too.

When Warren was in the sixth grade, he and his younger cousin, a third grader, were called to the administration office. A social worker was present and she asked questions about blood and bruises. Warren feared his grandmother's wrath and refused to tell the truth about them. His cousin, however, mentioned a couple of facts, but Warren remained silent and was released back to his classroom. Before Warren could complete elementary school at Balderas, he was moved to another school district after his grandmother moved the family to West Fresno. He would go on to finish the sixth grade at West Fresno Middle School, where it was combined with seventh and eighth graders.

While in the seventh grade in September of 2001, Warren hopped off the school bus, made the ten-minute walk home, and went into his grandmother's room to greet her. She was preoccupied on the phone discussing the news on the television. Warren fixated his eyes on her TV screen and watched as the twin World Trade Center towers in New York City collapsed. This was when Warren first got introduced to the term 'terrorism'. Schools and businesses continued to operate as usual while the country geared up for war against Al Qaeda. In December of 2001, however, Warren would experience another unexpected change in life. Grandma Peace had been sick her whole life and regularly made trips to the hospital, where she would spend nights at a time. The family was told she was to be released the following day. However, Aunt Rhonda, who came all the way from Stockton to watch over the house while her mother was in the hospital, barged in crying while Warren and his cousins slept, shouting that her mother was dead. Apparently, a nurse had come into Grandma Peace's room and saw her sitting upright with her head in her arm on her bedside table and pronounced her dead shortly after. On December 13, Grandma Peace passed away due to heart failure. Her children used the money she saved for her funeral, bought her a beautiful rosy pearl white coffin, and had her flown and laid to rest beside her mother, Madea, in Las Vegas, Nevada. The number thirteen would later stick out to Warren in adulthood because of the age difference between Samuel and his killer, the thirteen bullets that killed him, and because Warren was born thirteen years after his death in the same month Samuel was born – April.

Chapter III: Aunt Rhonda

After Grandma Peace's funeral, Warren wasn't given too many options on where he wanted to move or who he wanted to move in with. He also feared the wrong choice so he remained silent on the matter. Then, his Aunt Rhonda moved in, who was like her mother. She had a short temper, heavy hand, and could easily become aggravated or triggered. Warren didn't know much about his aunt other than her having lived in Stockton since he could remember and the fact she had a child named Georgia with a man who was incarcerated at the time. Aunt Rhonda was nice at first but authoritative. She also put Warren to a different kind of work than what he was used to. When she moved in and took over affairs after her mother passed, Aunt Rhonda began to remodel the place as if she owned it and Warren helped her every step of the way. It was a simple, three-bedroom rectangular-shaped house located on a corner across from a community park and multipurpose event center in West Fresno. They painted the walls, one of which was burnt orange. They tore up the old tiles throughout the house and replaced them with new ones. They planted flowers in the front yard and, in the backyard, was a pomegranate tree that constantly created a mess that Warren had to regularly keep clean.

On Warren's 12th birthday, Aunt Rhonda threw him a

party, had a bounce house set up in the backyard, and invited his cousins. Warren was having a decent time until he was made to clean the kitchen and guests' dishes in the middle of the event and then was dismissed early so the adults could have fun. Grownup's time meant for the aunts and uncles to get together to drink and smoke pot.

It was in that year Warren picked up an interest in the Harry Potter books. His Aunt Rhonda introduced him to the first movie, the Philosopher's Stone, but Warren has been addicted to reading the books ever since. He would lock himself in his room for hours at a time just to escape his world for a moment. At West Fresno Middle School, Warren entered a D.A.R.E. essay contest and placed first, winning multiple awards. He was at home; sick at the time and when he returned he was met with the news by his teacher, Mr. Clark. Warren liked this teacher. When he was sick, the teacher made the trip to his house in his mini SUV with 20'inch rims and hip hop music thumping from within to deliver homework he had missed while he was out.

At the end of the school year, Aunt Rhonda moved their little family to 128 San Joaquin street. This was the same house Warren lived in with his grandmother when he first came to Fresno six years earlier. He had lived in six or seven different homes since he last lived there. He begrudgingly moved back into the house where his abuse started. Also, Warren had to change schools again, this time to Fort Miller

Middle School near the Manchester Mall. One day, he missed his school bus and was too terrified to tell his aunt, but he did so anyway. She retaliated by having him clean the house on a time limit as if he was in Marine Corps boot camp. When he began to move too slow, she picked up a steel pot top and hit him with it. He had to clean each room this way. Also, Warren did not have room to call his own anymore as he personally felt his Aunt Rhonda loved to exercise her control over him. When they moved into the four-bedroom house, Warren was given one of the rooms in the back and then rotated between two others as the months passed for unknown reasons until he was placed into a make-shift den, which used to be the garage, and made to sleep there while there were other vacant rooms in the house. He could watch mice play with each other and zip back and forth in the dining room from where he used to lay in the den.

One late evening, on a school night, Warren got woken up abruptly by Aunt Rhonda and was made to come to her room. It was the house's biggest bedroom and was painted in a chipped sky blue. There was a large king mattress bed and frame in the middle, an old white vanity set with wig boxes and mannequin heads everywhere on shelves and on the floor. His aunt told him there was a bug that needed to be killed. Wondering why she couldn't do it, Warren looked for the insect and found it. When he quickly lost sight of it, his aunt snapped. She picked up a belt and began beating him with it. She yelled at him to get out, and he got back into his bed, his back became hot from her belt. About five minutes later, she barged in and ordered him to go back into her room and find the insect again. She threatened him with another beating. When he finally found the insect under one of her wigboxes in the corner of the room, he quickly grabbed his aunt's nearby ashtray, clenched it tight in his fist, and punched down on the insect, breaking the ashtray in his hand. The broken glass cut Warren's hand and he bled onto the floor. His aunt giggled nervously, told him to clean it, and get back to bed. Another night, Aunt Rhonda was in her bedroom again and she was upset about something he couldn't remember. When Warren didn't respond properly, she picked up a thick hangar and cracked him across the forehead with it. The strike sprouted a knot on his forehead that grew big and had a split. For parties or any events that Aunt Rhonda hosted, the guests found themselves disturbed by her treatment with Warren. One guest, a friend of the family, whom later Warren would grow to become fond of, recalled him being ordered around and treated as if he was his aunt's personal house slave. Warren lived in total fear and anxiety of his aunt and obeyed every one of her commands as if each word penetrated his soul and sought to break his spirit. He did as he was told and did not relent. He dared not to disrespect or further anger her despite the one time she yelled out, "I hate you!" He was doing his time. One month, Aunt Rhonda splurged on Warren, spending several hundred dollars on a new wardrobe. She was proud of it, even calling each of the family members to let them know and took pleasure in picking out each of his outfits each day before school. This bothered Warren deeply as it never allowed him to think for himself and practice independence. He felt it was another way for her to exercise control over his life. Aunt Rhonda bought him a Nintendo GameCube, which Warren loved. Playing video games presented another opportunity for Warren to leave his world for a time. However, within a couple of months of owning it, Aunt Rhonda said she needed to pawn it for money to buy marijuana. When she redeemed him on buying another GameCube several months later, it was sold again, this time for his Aunt Tania, who had come over one day claiming she needed money for gas.

Over the course of one summer, Warren was selected alongside a handful of students from his school to attend Fresno State University for a summer youth program. Warren enjoyed the program. Each day he went to school, he got onto another bus that took him and his summer classmates to the University in North Fresno. They'd attend classes, one of them dance and art, and then they'd have lunch at the dining commons. Warren loved the food and he could eat as much as he wanted. They'd finish out the day with one more class and then they'd take the bus back to Fort

Miller. Warren finished the summer program and had grown hopeful for his future and dreamed of college.

Aunt Rhonda loved Warren's hair. This was a total contrast to his grandmother, who disliked his hair and kept it shaven. His hair would grow exceptionally fast, thick, and could easily become wild. His aunt would tame it by braiding it. Her mood dictated how tight the braids were, and Warren dreaded it anytime she was in a bad one. One evening, she braided his hair so tight that Warren couldn't sleep. His Uncle Alfred, or Uncle 'Al', came and picked him up to hang out with him and his cousins over the weekend. Warren still couldn't sleep because of how tight the braids were. So, he took a pair of scissors and snipped the lower hairs above his neck to relieve the pressure that had been giving him headaches. A weekend later, Aunt Rhonda invited Aunt Tania's sons over to spend the night and redid Warren's hair. As she undid his braids, she noticed he had cut them. She snapped, hit and yelled at him in front of his cousins. When she was halfway through the redo, she sent him to a corner store with his two cousins to buy her a soda. While in the store, three young Hispanic girls about his age took notice of Warren, smiling at him. He kept to himself, filled the soda, and left the store with his cousins. When Warren stepped off the first curb, the soda slipped out of his hand and burst onto the street. He instantly knew another beating was coming his way. He had no money left and his aunt's soda cup was cracked. Before Warren could freak out, the three girls from the store approached them, and when they saw what had happened, they offered Warren their soda or money to replace it. Warren was grateful and smiled, but he declined their offer and returned home with his cousins to face the heat. To his surprise, Aunt Rhonda didn't hit him. She instead yelled at his mistake, gave him more money, sent him back to the store to get another soda and then finished his braids.

One day, Aunt Rhonda's boyfriend and father of her daughter, Demond, was released from prison. He had been serving time alongside Warren's dad, Dominic. They had even worked in the kitchen together. Warren didn't like Demond. Something of his vibes and energy rubbed him the wrong way. Demond didn't seem to be a fan of Warren either. Warren had heard stories of Demond and how he used to save his cousins from Aunt Rhonda's wrath. However, Warren never saw any such hero in him. If anything, Demond escalated tensions and the abuse further. Anytime Warren did anything, even if it was by mistake, Demond would alert Aunt Rhonda before she got home from work or school, and he'd have to hear her curses and threats with Demond sitting nearby with a smirk on his face. However, later, this couple began to steal. Warren would walk the halls in grocery stores and watch as Aunt Rhonda and Demond stole countless items ranging from electronics to household appliances. At a Walmart somewhere in Fresno County, Warren witnessed Aunt Rhonda and Demond walk right out the front door with two baskets full of goods. They then got into their car and left him at the store. While he was in the store, he could hear security describing his aunt's car and the direction it went. Aunt Rhonda and Demond later circled back and picked Warren up around the corner from the store. During the summer of that year, Aunt Rhonda picked up a job at a vacation park in Shaver Lake, cleaning the rental properties. She hadn't been there a month before she began loading her Ford Thunderbird up with furniture, appliances and food from each of the vacation homes she cleaned. Every day, Warren watched a new and used item fill their West Fresno home. Warren looked around at the new stuff and wondered if it meant a better life for them, or at the very least, for him. He wondered if the stealing would distract his aunt from beating him.

In the middle of the summer, Warren was sitting in the living room watching TV when his Aunt Rhonda rushed into the house, looking scared and worried. Warren had never seen her like this before. She looked incredibly nervous and told him and Georgia to go into her room, to wait there and not to come out until she asked them. They did as they were told. While Warren waited, he could hear her talk to Demond about a rifle, which he then took and dumped onto the side of the house. Within a few minutes, Warren could hear knocking on the front door. He heard the voices of police officers identifying themselves and then entering peacefully into the home. Warren didn't hear Aunt Rhonda or Demond say another word as they sat in the living room while the police roamed throughout the house. One of the officers, a white, blue-eyed male, found Warren in his aunt's room with his cousin. He said hello and introduced himself. Warren remembered him being nice and friendly. After a couple of minutes of waiting patiently, the officer asked Warren if he had seen anything new come into the house in recent weeks or if there was any suspicious activity with his aunt. Warren shook his head and said no. He dared not to say anything out of fear of his aunt. The officer politely waited for a few more moments before getting ready to leave the room. Warren's spirit was suddenly filled with fear, regret, and then ambition. He stopped the officer before he could leave and confessed what he had really seen, heard, and of the gun Demond dumped on the side of the house. The officer asked Warren if he knew anyone he wanted to pick him up. He asked for his Uncle Al, and he was there to take them to his home in the Tower District within the hour. The cops then hauled Aunt Rhonda and Demond to jail and Warren never lived with them again.

Chapter IV: The Tower District

Georgia was sent to Stockton to live with her father's parents until he and her mother could be released from jail. One of Warren's first acts since Aunt Rhonda's arrest was to have his hair cut. His Uncle Al took him to a barber and had his hair chopped off, leaving nothing but a curly afro. Then Warren settled in with his uncle at his small, one-bedroom apartment in the Tower District of Fresno. The district was known for its nightlife, having bars and many shops that line its main road on Olive Avenue and the historic Tower Theater on the corner of Wishon. Uncle Al lived in a rectangular apartment building South of Wishon, where it turns into North Fulton. The old building sat in between a business and a multiplex at the corner of North Fulton and Elizabeth. He had only lived in this apartment with his uncle for several months before they relocated a block away on Van Ness. However, before moving, Warren had to spend the rest of the summer in that small apartment with both of his uncle's sons, Benjamin and Christian, who had come down from Stockton to visit. Benjamin visited first, right after Warren settled. Out of the two brothers, Warren was most familiar with Benjamin. After Warren's mother died and Grandma Peace came to retrieve him from Stockton, they briefly stopped by Benjamin's mother's house, Serena, for a visit when she was still married to Uncle Al. Serena was also there for Warren's birth. That visit was the first time the two cousins had met, although they used to tot around Grandma Peace's house as toddlers when their parents briefly lived with her shortly after they were born. Benjamin admitted later that when he met Warren during that visit after Summer's death, he was terrified of him. The two had been born in the same year, two months apart, Benjamin in the middle of February and Warren in the middle of April. Perhaps this was another reason they remained so close throughout their teen years and adult life, more so than with any of their other cousins.

Benjamin could also, at times, come off as a little envious of Warren, perhaps because he got to live with his dad and was book-smart. Seldom they'd butt heads and get into a scuffle as most brothers do. However, one day, Warren and Benjamin got into a fight over a door. Benjamin had shoved a door onto Warren's foot, and he reacted by snapping and calling him a bitch. Aunt Tania, who lived over on Van Ness, had just visited with her two sons and overheard Warren shouting the curse. She beat him with a belt and that was the first time she ever hit him. Warren remembered this aunt as the one who would save him from Grandma Peace's beatings and would invite him out to lunch. The image he had of her being his favorite aunt had been shattered when she put a belt on his back. Benjamin would return home to Stockton, and his younger brother,

27

Christian, would take his place within a couple of weeks. Christian had been troubled, butting heads regularly with his mother, her new husband, and even his brother Benjamin. He had a bad habit of lashing out, stealing from his mother and stepdad, and fighting Benjamin. His mother had enough of Christian that summer and decided it was his turn to visit his father. At first, Christian appeared kind and Warren didn't understand what all of the fuss was about! However, one day, Warren rejected a sexual advance from him, and ever since, Christian retaliated by being a bully, even involving their other two cousins (Aunt Tania's sons) in the bullying. When it was announced that Christian's stay was going to be permanent and that they'd all soon have to move into Aunt Tania's two-bedroom apartment on Van Ness while she drove trucks across the region, he couldn't have felt any more troubled. He had escaped the wrathful abuse of his grandmother, then Aunt Rhonda's, and now he had to live with an emotionally disturbed aunt who would be gone for most of the weeks in a month, an uncle who had a drinking problem, and a handful of cousins who he felt envied, mocked, and hated him for reasons he wasn't too sure of.

Warren had known his Uncle Al to be an alcoholic and that he had troubles with the law prior to moving in with him. He remembered the day his uncle was released from prison and embraced Warren as if he had already known him. Ever since, Warren was fond of him. However, when they moved into Aunt Tania's apartment and she disappeared for weeks at a time for work Warren got to truly see his uncle for the person he had been so good at hiding from him and his cousins for so many years. This contrasted the uncle Warren thought he knew. The one that would gather the cousins together and even named them the Nephew Council. Of course, this would make his sons, Benjamin and Christian, envious, but when the group was together, they would go to the batting cages and movies, eat pizza, and have a sleepover at his apartment. They'd play games, listen to music, and watch sports. Everyone loved to escape the stress of their homes and hang out with Uncle Al. One evening, prior to moving over to Van Ness while Benjamin was still in town, he came in drunk. He was acting rude to Warren and even said some offensive comments like 'half-breed'. He pushed Warren and he pushed back. Uncle Al then grabbed Warren's head and slammed it onto the armrest of a chair in front of Benjamin and their cousins. A couple of days later, the cousins were play-wrestling and Benjamin, who liked to show out and impress others, especially with Warren as his guinea pig, took Warren and pedigreed him into the living room floor in front of Uncle Al, concussing him. Uncle Al said he would've stopped the action, but he thought his son was just playing around. Another evening, at the new apartment on Van Ness, Uncle Al barged in, ranting and raving about his night and then proceeded to insult each of his nephews when they didn't share his enthusiasm. When Warren responded in defense, his uncle hawked a big loogie onto his foot. Warren didn't speak to him the rest of the night. The next day, his uncle apologized to everyone, although Warren knew it wouldn't be the last time.

When Warren became a ninth grader in 2004, he got enrolled at Fresno High School. The administration gave his uncle his transcripts and when they got far enough from the school, his uncle showed him the spot on the document where it read that he sat in the top-six of his class. As for Christian, he was enrolled in a continuation school in West Fresno. While Uncle Al worked during the day and did school and the gym at night. Warren dealt with the bullying from his son and accomplices. Christian would ridicule, degrade, and at times try to fight Warren. When Warren tried to stand up for himself, Christian would retaliate with aggression. He would actively keep Aunt Tania's two sons involved in the bullying of Warren and there was never a day where he didn't feel as if something was being said behind his back or as if there was some plan to embarrass or demean him. Also, Christian loved to skip school, smoke pot, and steal money or bikes. These were the same reasons that got him kicked out of Stockton while living with his mother and stepdad. Warren, himself, started to steal candy from the Tower District's Dollar Tree store, rentable movies from

Blockbuster and even went as far as to swap out a busted Sony PlayStation Two with a working one at an old game store down the street from where they lived. When he succeeded with the last one, Christian found out and snitched him out to Aunt Tania. Infuriated, she walked Warren and his cousins to the game store to confirm him as the suspect so that she could beat him. The store owner's daughter, who was Hispanic and about Warren's age, had seen who took the game system and knew it was Warren, but when she saw him being led into the store and got asked if he was the one who did it, she shook her head no. Warren remembered Christian and their Aunt Tania's faces falling flat. He was surprised, too, but he dared not show it. He truly was appreciative of what that girl did. The owner dismissed Warren from the store and the others followed in silence all the way back to the apartment about a mile away. When they arrived, Aunt Tania apologized to Warren for accusing him and he couldn't have been any more grateful for that save. Warren remembered the days he'd follow Aunt Rhonda around the Food Maxx in West Fresno, and she'd swoop and steal as she turned each aisle, evading each camera as she went. He remembered on one of these trips, she brought Aunt Tania along and she partook in the activities. Warren couldn't believe the struggle was that bad, but it was.

***

When Benjamin came to visit during the winter holiday

break, he understood more than anyone how to both express his oppressive attitude toward others and how to deal with his brother's short-tempered, aggressive, and manipulative behavior. Christian managed to briefly persuade Benjamin into teaming up against Warren. However, when it became apparent that he was truly a bully and that Warren was already broken, he quickly became his ally. Perhaps some of Christian's actions also reminded Benjamin of what he went through in Stockton while living with him, but it became a regular habit for him to step in the middle of a rising fight between him and Warren. Anytime Christian cracked a degrading joke at Warren, Benjamin would counter it with one of his own. When Christian tried to pick a fight and even tried to swing at Warren, Benjamin would intervene and resort to fighting him instead, throwing fists. Warren knew it was a matter of time before Benjamin had to go back home to Stockton, which he eventually did once his break ended, but they grew exceptionally close ever since. One evening, Warren finally decided to file a formal complaint to his uncle, but he refused to listen. His uncle was in his room, lying on his bed, wearing the beanie he usually wore when he slept. Warren told him what happened when he wasn't around, and he shrugged him off, barely saying two words.

Warren left his room and went into the one he shared with Christian and the other two cousins. It was empty except for the long wraparound couch they all used as a bed.

Warren turned out the light and his body froze in place. He couldn't understand what was happening. His head tilted to the right and he began to gasp. The room was pitch dark and he felt trapped in his body, unable to escape the terror trickling down his spine. Then, he was allowed to inhale a breath of air and he snapped out of his bind. He flipped the light on, swung the door open, and ran out into the hall, terrified. His cousins were watching TV and his uncle was still in his room. He tried to tell someone but was ignored. When Warren went to bed that night, he experienced sleep paralysis for the first time. As he descended into sleep, his body froze while his mind stayed awake. He would hallucinate in the dark, hearing what sounded like a jet airplane engine, powered on as if in a testing hangar and it being lowered on top of him. Every night ever since, Warren struggled to sleep and would continue to experience these events for the next fourteen years.

***

One day, Christian needed to do something for school downtown and asked his dad if someone could go with him, so Warren was sent. They barely spoke to each other on the bus ride to the main transportation hub at the county courthouse to switch routes. They got off the first bus and they had only been waiting about five minutes for their next bus to arrive when two African American boys ran in from out of nowhere and got in Christian's face. The boys were much bigger than both Christian and Warren and the main antagonist was ready to fight. He asked Christian, "So, what was all that stuff you were saying back at school? What are you going to do now? What are you going to say now?" He had his fists up, rocking them back and forth, ready to tango. Warren has never seen Christian so unsure of what to do. He clearly did not want to fight. If anything, Christian looked intimidated. Warren, without properly thinking but going with the spark that had just filled his chest, stepped in between Christian and the two boys. "Back off of my cousin," he said, not entirely thinking. "Or you're going to have to fight me." He couldn't believe he was defending this asshole cousin. To his surprise, the boys couldn't believe it either. They backed away, relented, and told Christian they'd see him around. They left the hub as Warren and Christian boarded their bus. Later that night, Christian hurried to tell everyone what happened that day, probably to beat Warren to the storytelling. In Christian's version, he tried to say even if Warren had fought them, he would've got beaten up. But, the cousins who heard the story respected and treated Warren positively ever since and Christian retaliated. A night or so later, a scuffle ensued between Christian and one of the cousins and Warren had to intervene. Christian lost a game of Yu-gi-oh and in the act of poor sportsmanship, tried to choke out his cousin. His cousin looked up at Warren with tears in his eyes and asked for him to get Christian off him.

One morning, Warren set out for school, walking to Fresno High as he usually did. The walk usually took anywhere from 15-20 minutes. He had just barely crossed into the block adjacent to his and made a turn onto the empty and semi-vacant street when an old, light-colored compact car being driven by an Asian, most likely Chinese, pulled up beside him. The man inside had long, straight black hair that lay flat on both sides of his head and wore a white t-shirt. He asked Warren if he could do him a favor and come with him so that he could knock on his girlfriend's door for him. The man pointed to a nearby apartment building across the vacant lot across the street that Warren recognized as his uncle's old building on North Fulton before they moved over to Van Ness. Warren knew the man was lying and his every nerve told him to keep saying, "No." After the third no, the man sped off and Warren picked up a thick branch and carried it with him the rest of the way to school. He told his uncle when he got home later that day and Uncle Al was furious. He lectured the cousins that evening and told family members what had happened.

It was around this time, while in a Fresno High science class, Warren discovered he had a passion for saving animals. His teacher would regularly, usually once a month, feed a rat from the pet store to the class's pet snake. The snake would wrap its body around the poor little prey, squeeze the life out of it, and then swallow him whole.

Warren was already familiar with the feeding process, having watched a film called Anaconda while living with Aunt Rhonda. The teacher brought a fresh rat to class, threw him into the snake's aquarium, and everyone waited until it would get devoured. However, the snake didn't eat him right away and Warren knew he had to save him. So, when class ended, Warren exited out one of the doors that led straight outside instead of into the building's interior hall and asked his Hispanic friend, Eddie, to hold the door for him and be a lookout while he rescued the rat. Eddie agreed and posted as a lookout. Warren ran inside and, with a lunch box he had found in a trash can outside the classroom, scooped the rat out of the aquarium and put him inside and then into his backpack. He fled the classroom, thanked Eddie, and went home. He showed the rat to his uncle and cousins, who all found his story to be amusing. He named the rat 'Scabbers' after the one in Harry Potter. Uncle Al took him to the pet store several months later and bought him a female rat. He named her 'Cecilia'. The two birthed about six baby mice and then Scabbers died shortly afterward. Warren and his cousins loved playing the trading card game, Yu-gi-oh. They'd regularly make bets for each other's cards; in this case, Christian put in a bet for one of Warren's mice. So, they battled it out over the ownership of one of them. Although Warren could have beaten Christian with the hand, he had. He lost on purpose so that he could have a pet.

Before Grandma Peace died three years earlier, Warren's Uncle Victor, the one he feared the most, moved his family to Jackson, Mississippi. His family consisted of himself, his wife, and six girls, two of which were his by blood. Perhaps life was difficult for them there, or maybe word of what took place at Aunt Tania's apartment when neither she nor Uncle Al were around got back to him, but Uncle Victor decided to move back to California with his family sometime after his mother's death. Aunt Tania permitted them to live in her two-bedroom apartment with everyone else until they could find a place of their own. So, Warren waited until the day for the uncle, who terrified him and took pleasure in beating him in the name of Grandma Peace, could move in. Even Christian feared Uncle Victor. The only positive Warren saw at first with his uncle moving in was that Christian would be too scared to do any of his usual antics. Warren and his male cousins slept in the living room as their bedroom was taken over by their uncle. It was an old, vintage building, and every creak, step, and flush could be easily heard. Christian used to make matters worse when he would jump up and down on the living room floor in response to banging on the ceiling from the neighbors below them.

One midday, Uncle Al burst into the apartment drunk off whiskey. As usual, he began dishing out insults and he called Warren a half-breed as usual. Warren responded by saying, "Fuck you, bitch!" and his uncle, always the prideful type, punched Warren squarely in the chest, making him double over. This strike made Warren remember an earlier time when his grandma Peace was alive and Uncle Al's sons had come to visit. He remembered his uncle and cousins taking turns on who could humiliate Warren first. One time, in the hallway of his grandma's apartment at Maple Grove, when Warren was about eight years old, his uncle hit him in the chest and made him lose his breath for unknown reasons to him. His cousins laughed at him, and Warren didn't understand why his uncle, who was his favorite, betrayed him unexpectedly like that. Now, nearly six years later, he finally understood. His uncle was truly an alcoholic. So, Warren took the blow, but this time he stormed off out the back door, furious. On his way down the stairs, he saw Uncle Victor sitting on one of the lower steps smoking a cigarette. He blew past him and ran for the corner of the yard where he had buried Scabbers about a month or so earlier. Uncle Victor followed him, put out his cigarette, and approached him cautiously. "What's wrong?" he asked. Warren waited and wondered how best to respond to him. He decided to leave out what he said that escalated the interaction with Uncle Al and instead listed everything wrong his uncle did prior to cursing at him. "Uncle Al came in drunk," Warren said. "Called me a half-breed and then hit me in the chest." Uncle Victor didn't say another word to Warren. He turned on his heel, stormed up the stairs, and burst into the

38

apartment. Warren could hear shouts and threats. When his uncle came back down, he apologized for his brother's actions and told him if anyone did something like that to him again, to let him know. Warren nodded his head in agreement and his uncle left. Later that evening, right before dinner, Uncle Victor sat with Warren in the backyard and apologized for what he did to him while Grandma Peace was alive. He explained that he did it for her and that he had become a better person since. Warren couldn't believe they were even having that conversation. He never knew Uncle Victor was capable of apologizing. Warren, without thinking about it, forgave him.

About a month later, toward the end of that summer in 2005, an eviction notice was served due to noise and overcrowding. Everyone would have to split up and find their own way. So, plans were made and one-way bus tickets were purchased. Aunt Tania and her two sons relocated to an apartment next to Fresno State University, Uncle Victor and his family moved to an apartment in Central Fresno, and Uncle Al, before moving in with a close friend, put Warren and Christian on a greyhound. The plan was for Warren to stay at his Aunt Serena's house in Stockton until summer ended and then return to Fresno. However, Warren had no intention of returning.

Chapter V: Stockton

Aunt Serena and her husband received Warren warmly. He liked his aunt, she was always much nicer than his blood relatives, and anytime Warren used to visit, he thought hanging out with this family was one of his favorite things to do. After a couple of weeks, his aunt asked if he wanted to live with them permanently because there was nowhere else for him to go if he were to go back to Fresno. He said yes and they allowed him to stay.

Warren was enrolled in Bear Creek High School but was only there a semester before the family moved, and he had to transfer to Stagg High, where Benjamin attended. He was only there for a semester as well before having to transfer to Cesar Chavez High due to another residential move. It was at Cesar Chavez that Warren excelled in his grades, achieving membership in the National Society of High School Scholars, in Who's Who Among American High School Students, and received many other awards and recognitions such as Honor Roll and Perfect Attendance. As he walked the halls one day, a football coach approached him, fascinated by his size. Warren had reached an age in which he began to grow taller, bigger, and his voice began to deepen. People began to assume he was a Samoan because of how big he began to look. The coach encouraged him to try out, and Warren did, but the family moved again.

Therefore, so did he. He transferred schools again, this time to Ronald E. McNair High. This was around the time that Christian began to lash out again. He had been doing it sporadically since they moved to Stockton, but Warren began to see what got him kicked out in the first place. He began stealing money from his mother again, her bikes, and countless other items from around the house. He also hung around the wrong crowds and got into a lot of fights at home and outside of it. Benjamin had to wrestle with him a couple of times, and one day, he tried to pick a fight with Warren with Benjamin and Aunt Serena's husband as witness. Christian had poked Warren's face, and in an instant, he lifted Christian off his feet, body-slammed him, and gave him one good punch to the ribcage. Christian never messed with Warren again. Christian would eventually find himself getting locked up in the juvenile hall and spending time in all-boys camps.

***

In the mid of 2007, the family moved to a cul-de-sac to a little brown house where Aunt Serena's mother-in-law used to live. When her mother-in-law moved into a bigger house, Aunt Serena and her husband moved in and took over affairs. It was in this cul-de-sac where Warren befriended two neighborhood boys who also attended the same school at McNair High. They'd walk to school together, hang out on campus, and when school was over, they'd walk back to their court. One day, while the three were hanging out around the neighborhood, one of the friends presented the idea that he'd been discussing with the other to Warren. The plan was to form a clique and give it a name. Warren agreed to it and said they would need to get jumped in before they could join and become official members. So, they each stood still, taking turns hitting each other in the upper arms until they bruised and felt sore. Their group became official and they continued to hang out as usual with plans to expand. Then, Warren's grades began to decline. One day, after school, Warren watched as his two friends antagonized and tried to fight a student who was walking home with his little brother. Nothing happened, but Warren knew it was wrong. About a week later, Benjamin told his parents what Warren had done and they confronted him about it. Aunt Serena's husband had a bad habit of communicating in a way that was aggressive and he enjoyed poking fun at Warren in front of people. Warren didn't understand why people liked to mess with him in front of other people. He was outside washing his aunt's car and his friends were nearby. His aunt's husband came out after he heard that Warren had joined a clique and took the water hose from him and began squirting him with it in front of everyone. Warren was baffled. He stood there getting soaked and his friends knew it angered him. They remained silent and watched as Warren got in his uncle's face, grabbed the water hose, and told him if he squirted him again, he was going to fight him in the street. Benjamin was also nearby and started laughing. Warren, knowing his aunt's husband wasn't going to fight him, turned his attention to Benjamin. He saw his cousin's big pre-workout supplement jug on the ground and picked it up. Warren busted it on the ground, and the powder scattered and blew into the wind. "That's for laughing," Warren told Benjamin and went inside. The next day, Aunt Serena picked Warren up from school and asked if he was really going to fight her husband. He said yes because he felt he had been humiliated. When they got to the house, she told Warren he'd have to go back to Fresno. Warren couldn't believe it. He figured it was because he wasn't their blood relative, but he wasn't given a fair defense. He agreed to leave anyway and didn't say another word. They put Warren on a greyhound that evening and sent him back to Fresno.

Chapter VI: Fresno

It had only been a year and a half since Warren left Fresno for Stockton after they got evicted and he couldn't believe he was already coming back. His stupid mistakes got him sent back to a place he dreaded and had a stressful and traumatic history in. When he arrived at the greyhound station late at night, his Uncle George was waiting for him in his work truck. Warren didn't mind this uncle even though he, too, can become temperamental and controlling. He had heard a story of this uncle when he was growing up of how he was sitting on the hood of a car when he was a teen and fell off. They said he hit his head and died, and the doctors brought him back to life. Ever since, he's been quick-tempered, impulsive, and into his vices. When he picked Warren up, he barely said two words to him. Warren already knew and felt he was not wanted. He had no choice but to choose this uncle. He never spoke to Uncle Victor, hadn't said two words to Aunt Tania since he last lived with her, and his Uncle Al was serving time for driving while intoxicated. While Warren was living in Stockton with Aunt Serena, word got to him from Fresno that Uncle Al had been over at a family friend's drinking excessively. He then got into his Ford Probe and had one of Aunt Tania's sons with him. While on a curved high-rise freeway, Uncle Al fell asleep, and his car veered off the bridge and vaulted into the air, flipping downhill as it crashed. They survived, but Uncle Al broke his leg, got air-lifted to a hospital, and then got thrown in jail. Uncle George dropped Warren off at his apartment in the ghetto in Central Fresno and left to work for his overnight shift at his security job. Warren settled into the shared bedroom with Uncle George's two sons and fell asleep. When he woke up the next day, his uncle was in the living room smoking pot. He told him to explain what happened in Stockton and Warren did. His uncle asked him if he smoked pot and he said no. He then dismissed him to the bedroom. He now shared a room with his cousins. Warren found himself, even though at the age of seventeen, having to remain in the bedroom with his two cousins until his uncle told them they could come out.

Warren got re-enrolled at Fresno High, where his cousin, George Jr., also attended. This was the same cousin who slipped facts about the abuse going on at home when they were called in to speak with a social worker at Balderas Elementary. They'd take the city bus back and forth to campus. Warren picked up an elective as a library assistant, and after only a month of working there, he was called into the head librarian's office. She was a kind Hispanic lady and showed him a paid job posting. It was for a kitchen assistant position.

Warren thanked her and said he'd apply. He took the city bus after school to meet the hiring manager, and when he arrived, he was surprised to discover it was a Fresno State University sorority house. A couple of houses away from the Bulldog Football Stadium, Warren met with an elderly kitchen lady named Sally. She hired Warren on the spot, and he started cleaning and tidying as he went. She gave him a plate of food and sent him away to return the next day. She did this almost every night. Warren liked his first job, he always maintained respect and did as he was told. He helped Sally make dinners every night for the house tenants and events. He'd prep, clean, close, and then take the 30-minute bus ride back to Uncle George's. When he received his first check, he created a bank account and reimbursed his uncle for the bus fare he had to borrow to get to work each day. He was surprised to find that his uncle wanted more of the check. His uncle even went as far as to calculate everything Warren had been using up to that point in terms of food, resources, and even the bus fare. Warren was taken aback. He offered to give his uncle more money, but his uncle refused him. The next day, Warren contacted his Aunt Tania, who still lived next to Fresno State with her family as well as the sorority house where he worked, and asked to move in with her. She agreed, and Warren packed up his belongings from his uncle's apartment and moved out. Although this aunt was no longer his favorite, Warren felt she was the last option in town. When she received him, he felt he had to force a smile and pretend he still valued her the same. She now had a baby daughter plus her two sons and was unemployed at that time. Warren moved into the shared boys' room and was mentally prepared to graduate from high school and move on in life. In that winter of 2007, Warren requested to graduate a semester early due to high credits and it was granted. Because he was no longer a student, his employment at the Fresno State sorority house had to end, and through the end of winter and into the spring of 2008, he would work direct sales for a security alarm company based in North Fresno, making a lot of commission. Warren disliked his second job after the sorority house. He had to work with unethical people who liked to sleep with each other despite the fact they had significant others at home. He also had a supervisor who liked to sexually harass women everywhere they wentand would eventually get terminated due to his harassment of a new hire who was going through orientation. This supervisor also tried to take a verbal jab at Warren one day while at lunch before they were to set out across the county to knock on doors. He overheard Warren tell an interested coworker that he was planning on going to college after he stopped working with them and that he wanted to produce films and other forms of entertainment. The supervisor interrupted and told Warren he would never succeed in such a thing and then resumed eating once everyone fell silent at the table. Warren kept his distance ever since from the supervisor and would only remain at the company until the week of his 18th birthday in the middle of April. In the last couple of weeks leading up to his birthday, however, Warren would get bitten by a dog while working, would see his coworkers' personal relationships get shattered by their work relationships, and would lose his direct supervisor due to sexual harassment. His head boss also borrowed money from him and never paid it back. Meanwhile, his relationship with his Aunt Tania was straining again as she began to demand more of him each day. She told Warren he needed to find another job as she didn't consider it reliable, that it didn't pay well enough, and that she needed him to support her and her kids. Warren didn't understand her angle. He couldn't believe what she said to him. He was not her husband and surely was not there to support her or her family. He was there temporarily as a stepping block to get to where he needed to go in life. What made matters worse was that, while tensions were rising at Warren's toxic work environment, he'd have to come home and deal with his aunt breathing down his neck the moment he walked in the door. As soon as he made a mess, she barked for it to be cleaned and kept him on what felt like a tight schedule. Warren was not sure what her deal was. Knowing he needed an outlet and knowing that his general manager had an extra room at his apartment in Central Fresno, Warren paid his boss for a week's stay until he could extend with the next paycheck. On the last night of living with his Aunt Tania, Warren walked into the apartment and it was quiet except for the humming of the dishwasher. The overhead stove light was on and Warren used it to make Top Ramen noodles. He had barely spilled crumbs onto the counter when his aunt walked in and snapped. "If you can't follow the rules, then you are going to need to leave," she said.

That was all Warren needed to hear. He had enough of her controlling tendencies and her overbearing and micromanaging behaviors and attitudes. He was done. "Okay, I will leave," Warren said humbly, wiping his hands together. He went into the room he shared with his cousins and his aunt followed. He began packing his stuff, shoving his clothes into a single duffle bag.

"What are you doing?", Aunt Tania asked, wide in the eyes.

"Leaving," Warren replied. "Since I am not following your rules as you say, I am leaving. Bye."

Aunt Tania didn't utter another word to Warren. She got on the phone and began crying to another relative and ordered one of her sons to follow Warren around to make sure he didn't steal anything. This cousin didn't listen and understood what Warren had to do. He even defended Warren after he left. When Warren got married twelve years later, this cousin served as his best man. Warren called a yellow cab and for the first time in his life, he left his family. When he arrived at his boss' apartment, which sat in a rough neighborhood in Central Fresno, he was surprised to find that no one was home. With the door locked, lights off, and it being late into the evening, Warren set up camp outside on the apartment's stairwell and fell asleep.

Chapter VII: Coming of Age

It was around this time in the middle of April, during the week of Warren's 18th birthday, that he smoked tobacco for the first time. He bought a pack of cigarillos from a corner store near his boss' apartment complex and smoked each one down until a coworker of his, who was also staying with their boss for some time, convinced him to calm down. Warren didn't like this coworker much. He, too, was temperamental and occasionally butted heads with Warren everywhere they went and when he didn't get his way. Warren could never shake him off. They used to walk to work together as they used to live in the same neighborhood near Fresno State and would hitch rides together. One time, this coworker wanted the front seat of another coworker's car even though Warren called it first and took it. The coworker, whom he didn't care much for, tried to rear choke him from the back seat until Warren repelled him. Ever since Warren despised him. When Warren moved into his boss' apartment a day or so later, he found out this troubled coworker was going to move in, too. It reminded Warren of when he lived with his Uncle Al and then with his Aunt Serena. No matter where he went during those years, his annoying and tyrannical cousin Christian had to move with him too. After a couple of days of living with his boss and coworker, Warren called his Aunt Serena in Stockton. He was glad to hear her voice despite how their last conversation ended. He apologized for how things played out when he lived with her and asked for forgiveness. She forgave him instantly and they made arrangements for him to get picked up by Benjamin. Warren didn't announce the news to his boss and coworkers until the next day, hours before Benjamin was set to pick him up. He knew he'd hear resistance. Warren was used to people trying to hold other people back; surely, that is what they tried to do. When Warren told his general manager he no longer needed to extend his stay with him while at a team meeting, his boss' face fell. He tried to convince Warren that moving back in with his family was a bad idea and that he should try to become an adult and find his own way. Warren said he felt confident in what he was doing and then spent the remainder of the shift dreading each passing minute that he had to endure with them. Benjamin arrived in his parents' white Ford Expedition with Bob, his white best friend and their former neighbor. Warren snatched his bag out of one of the company vans and hurried to them. When Benjamin saw a pack of cigarillos in Warren's hand, he took them and hurled the box over the fence in the company parking lot and they landed in a pond. Warren smiled and hopped in the Expedition as his former coworkers looked on. He left Fresno and would never live there again.

***

When they arrived in Stockton, Warren was eased back

into normal without too much conflict. He was warned that certain aggressive behaviors wouldn't be tolerated and they hoped to move forward from it. A month after he turned eighteen, Warren enlisted in the United States Marine Corps. Benjamin had already gone and graduated while Warren lived in Fresno the last several months, following somewhat in the footsteps of his father Al, who served twenty years earlier. Warren needed a path to help him transition into adulthood as he didn't have any positive adult role models around. Although he aspired to attend college one day, he felt joining the military was something that couldn't wait. A month after enlisting and getting sworn in at the Sacramento MEPS, Warren shipped off for a three-month boot camp at the MCRD in San Diego, one month of combat school at Camp Pendleton, and three months of occupational specialty school at Camp Johnson in North Carolina. It was through this training cycle, in combination with his age and experiences that Warren further adopted quick-tempered, retaliatory, and obsessive-compulsive type tendencies.

While in boot camp in Southern California, he'd butt heads with fellow recruits, get into a couple of scuffles, and he shoulder-checked a kill-hat drill instructor on his way into the House of Knowledge. The kill-hat tried to punish Warren at the obstacle course and dirt pit across the street for it, but he got saved by his senior-drill instructor at the last second, who told him to hurry up and get inside.

Another day, while out on the shooting range, his junior-hat drill instructor accused Warren of pointing his weapon at him. Warren didn't do such a thing and he felt the drill instructor set it up to have him verbally blasted in front of the entire company. A group of drill instructors circled Warren because of this accusation, and they all shouted and humiliated him in front of his peers. Warren was never so angry about getting punished for a lie. He would later discover the other drill instructors, behind the scenes, would talk smack and pick on the junior-hat instructor who accused Warren of flagging him with his gun.

Another day, a white recruit was sitting on Warren's foot locker. Warren told him to get off and he refused even though there was a clear rule set to never sit on the lockers. Warren snatched the recruit into a headlock, and before fists could be thrown, it was broken up.

Later that night, Warren swapped his own name out on the fire watch schedule with the recruit he had wrestled with earlier in the day. Warren was caught the next day, and when he confessed and explained to his senior-drill instructor, who was also white, why he did it, he went unpunished. If anything, the senior-drill instructor thought it was amusing. Warren would later come to love boot camp. It was the one time in his life he got to let off steam by screaming and yelling at the top of his lungs, running across California's Southern hills with full gear, and shooting relentlessly on the ranges. Warren loved to shoot and was good at it. He would test out as an expert rifleman, but he enjoyed any weapon he managed to get his hands on. Also, he had lost a lot of weight. He had been getting made fun of for getting thicker over the recent years, but since he began training with the Marines, he shredded weight like none other and began to find the foundation for his new look.

Warren loved the scenery of North Carolina when he got sent there for motor transport maintenance school at Camp Johnson near Camp Lejeune. He would eventually have to return to it for another three months for an advanced motor course, but each time he stayed, he loved the greenery, the flat roads, the architecture of its brick homes, and how differences in culture it was in comparison to California. He even got to touch the Atlantic Ocean when he took a trip with a hometown friend to Myrtle Beach, South Carolina, over one liberty weekend. One cold, snowy evening while doing fire watch on base. Warren passed a barracks room and the door swung open. Some Marines, all of them white, had been drinking and were arguing. Warren, in his big-boy Marine voice, told them to settle down. One of the Marines turned and called him a nigger. The other white Marines didn't laugh or budge. If anything, they looked surprised their roommate even said it. Up to that point, Warren had never really been called the n-word with the hard-R, perhaps because of his light-brown and yellowish complexion. It had mostly been said in passing as a joke amongst family members and friends at school. Warren was most familiar with the Asian population in Stockton and how they loved to use the relaxed-A version at a higher frequency than any other race he had ever known. Some of the Asians in Stockton, a town they have a historical majority in, adopted the word and applied it to their hip-style and culture, so to Warren, it became very common to hear it. That was Stockton's culture and Warren was used to it. So, when the racist cast his insult, Warren laughed in his face. The Marine did not say another word, and Warren continued with his patrol, not saying another word to him. While still in North Carolina that winter over the holiday break because he did not want to visit California or anyone there for that matter, Warren had the pleasure of speaking with his Uncle Curt over the phone, who was the oldest of Grandma Peace's children. After a long life of living on the west coast, Uncle Curt picked up his family and moved to Florida. Warren heard stories of this uncle when he was living with his grandmother. How he rebelled against his mother's abuse, and when she tried to stop him from leaving when he turned eighteen, he told her he was too old for it and was done with her matriarchy. She let him go and he never returned. He would get married, have children, and remain distant from his family until he was able to physically move as far away as he was in spirit from them. It was for about two hours when he called and spoke with Warren in North Carolina. He told Warren everything; how he left the family to save himself, how he disliked his sister Rhonda because of her aggressive attitude, and how when Grandma Peace died, he wanted to adopt Warren but couldn't due to the family rejecting his requests. For their two-hour conversation, Warren realized that this uncle would have been his favorite rather than Uncle Al had things been different. Finally, Warren thought, he had an uncle, a family member who understood what he went through because he, too, went through the same traumas and sought to be different and get better from it. Warren graduated from his military occupational school in North Carolina in the middle of February, 2009. In June of that year, he received a call saying his Uncle Curt had passed away due to heart failure. It was the same condition with Grandma Peace succumbed to eight years prior. The only person Warren felt he could relate to in his family was gone. He didn't get to go to his uncle's funeral in Florida, but a couple of his close relatives did. Warren heard that Aunt Rhonda attended and made a fool of herself in front of everyone at the funeral by being loud and obnoxious, thus disrespecting Uncle Curt's wife and son. Uncle Curt's family hasn't spoken to the rest of the Peace family since that day, Warren included.

When Warren returned to Stockton after his military training, he moved into a shared duplex with Benjamin. For a brief period, Christian was released from one of his detention camps. He had gotten reacquainted with old friends and asked Warren for a ride to one of their homes. Warren dropped him off later that day and randomly talked with a white male police officer while waiting in line at a Starbucks. Later in the week, on the same street of that Starbucks, called Pacific Ave. Warren saw this same officer again when he got pulled over for what he first thought was a regular traffic stop for having his cellphone to his ear. He had been making a U-turn in his 1996 Acura Integra onto Pacific Ave, going north toward the malls when he noticed a squad car tailing him. Suddenly, more squad cars raced forward and veered in front of his car, preventing him from driving further. Warren stopped the car, turned it off, and did everything as he was told. He had a baby cousin inside and was told to walk back to the officers who had guns pointed at him. So, Warren walked backward, got put in handcuffs, and was put into the back of a squad car. One of the officers told him he was going to retrieve his identification from the car and Warren didn't argue. When the officer returned to go through his wallet, he was surprised to find a military ID card inside. Another officer, whom Warren had recognized as the one he spoke to in the Starbucks line a few days prior, walked up to the others to look at the identification cards. He frowned when he saw Warren's face in the photos and raised his eyebrows when he looked Warren in the eyes. He quickly told the other officer they had the wrong guy. The officers corrected themselves and let Warren out of the car, freed him from his cuffs, and spoke with him respectfully, explaining they were searching for his cousin, Christian. They told him an eyewitness saw Warren's car drop off a suspect in a neighborhood where a crime was committed. Warren told the officers he didn't know where his cousin was, and after returning his property, they kindly let him go.

***

Warren had worked odd jobs for two years since he came back from North Carolina, and in the fall of 2010, he applied for freshman admission into San Jose State University.

He was provisionally accepted and made plans to leave Stockton and the Great Central Valley for good. He made a deal with his Aunt Serena's husband to switch him vehicles for a year until he settled in his new home. Her husband agreed, and Warren traded him a lifted, black mid-90s Chevy Tahoe for a 2002 white, standard Dodge Ram pickup truck.

Using a social media school group page, Warren found roommates and a two-bedroom townhouse for them to share in Japantown in San Jose, about a mile north of campus. Warren had attended a new student event over the summer and applied to the campus dining commons. He got the job and received a call from the head chef asking if he wanted to start the week before school began. He accepted, loaded his belongings into the Ram, and moved into the townhouse earlier than the other roommates. He began his duties at the dining commons prepping meals for faculty, athletes, and events. He was glad. By this point, rumors had been circulating that new students were being dropped before school started and would continue to do so through the first week of classes. The reasons were errors on transcripts or misreported grades. Warren remembered this causing a stir and a frenzy within the freshman population. No one knew who would get dropped and many were getting dropped at a high rate. People threatened the school with lawsuits, parents called admissions to appeal, and students emotionally collapsed in shame. Warren didn't expect to get dropped, but when he received a letter after the first week of classes saying his admission into the school had been revoked, he thought his life was over. He felt horrified and a failure. Everything was tied into the school and now that he was no longer a student. He expected everything to fall through and move back to Stockton. He refused to go back to that shithole. His aunt Serena and her husband were going to help ensure that didn't happen either.

After everything he had been through with his blood relatives, he was now at odds with Benjamin's Mother and Stepdad again, but this time over the truck swap, he never bothered to get in writing. While Warren had been dealing with the failures of getting revoked from school, his fake aunt's husband sold the Tahoe, kept the profits, and now wanted the Ram returned. Warren was distraught. He tried to fight it, argued, and when he utterly refused to return the vehicle until he got another one or at least the money from the Tahoe sale, his aunt called the San Jose Police Department and reported the vehicle stolen. She also got his Aunt Rhonda involved. The investigating officer told them he didn't want to ruin Warren's life over a family dispute when he had a clean record. Aunt Rhonda then acted, texting and calling Warren in the name of Aunt Serena. She ordered him to give her back the truck and he felt she was trying to use fear to get him to obey. They were teaming up against him. He couldn't believe it. Warren flipped and then snapped. He told his Aunt Rhonda to mind her own damn business, called her every bad name and slander in the devil's black book, and then commanded her to never speak to him again. For the first time in his life, he got to tell his aunt what he really thought of her. She didn't say a word back and he hung up. The next day, after a night of pondering, Warren parked the truck near the airport and they came and retrieved it. Once the dust settled, Warren turned his attention to his Aunt Serena and called the government agency she had been defrauding. For two years, she had been falsely using his name for child care benefits for two years. She made Warren pose as a babysitter for her children so that he could receive extra money her actual babysitter had rejected. As planned, she began receiving monthly checks that were in Warren's name and deposited them into a bank account that she had convinced him to start with her.

Warren called the agency she had been defrauding and filed a claim. About a month later, Aunt Serena and a couple of others from her extended family, whom Warren was much fond of, came to San Jose to have lunch with him. Aunt Serena appealed to Warren and asked if he could reverse what he told the investigators. After much reluctance, Warren agreed, but under the condition that she finds him a vehicle to replace the one that was stolen from him. She reached out to Benjamin for one of his vehicles and he sent him a brown 2000 Grand Jeep Cherokee. She never received another check from that agency and Warren ceased communications with her and her family.

Chapter VIII: San Jose

Warren started smoking again, this time cigarettes. He also began to drink and party, spending most of his weekly money on parties. He also picked up membership at a local mixed martial arts and kickboxing gym called Tribull and then remained a member for a brief time when it merged with Dark Horse. He had already achieved a gray belt in Marine Corps martial arts, but he trained, achieved belts in Kajukenbo, gained further confidence in himself and his kickboxing, and ground fighting capabilities. Meanwhile, in the military, Warren had transferred his home reserve unit from Sacramento to San Jose when he moved for school. However, rather than the Sacramento administration clerk doing a successful inter-unit transfer, he instead dropped Warren to the inactive-ready reserve. This meant Warren had to no longer drill once a month and his benefits would cease. He was out of his military contract three years earlier than expected. In addition to that error, communication wasn't passed properly up the chain of command when Warren told leadership in Sacramento that he was cleared to transfer and would be doing so immediately. Instead, Warren was reported as an unauthorized absence or U.A. This disqualified him from his education and other military benefits, and he was no longer allowed to receive the reserve-G.I. bill. When the transfer was corrected, Warren called his former Sacramento unit to have his benefits restored, and the gunnery sergeant said that by the time it got fixed, he would be out of the military. This further depressed and demoralized Warren and sent him down a brief spiraling path of drunkenness, smoking tobacco, and acting like a belligerent fool in the community. His behavior became turbulent. He'd do silly things like climb a railroad track's signal arms with housemates and get the cops called on him. He'd also blurt the first thing that would come to his mind, he'd explode and erupt in anger when someone offended him, and he'd invade people's personal spaces to disrupt them anytime he felt they did something that posed as a trigger to him. At sporting events, he'd act out like a drunkard for attention and would embarrass his roommates with his aggressive and buffoonish behaviors. One day, his roommates were smoking marijuana in the house, and he took the joint from them and threw it off the second-floor balcony. He'd regularly have power-play and controlling tendencies within the townhouse he shared with his three housemates. Everyone had to clean up after themselves, everything had to be kept clean, and anytime someone didn't follow a house rule, there was a good chance they were going to hear from Warren about it.

Warren remained working at the campus dining commons despite no longer being a student. This wasn't much of a problem, he thought, as there were several others who were working there as non-students as well. Refusing to fall behind those he moved to San Jose with, Warren signed up for film school at the Academy of Art University in San Francisco. He had done a couple of online classes with them the year before he moved out of Stockton but discontinued them when he got accepted into SJSU. The Academy of Art accepted him back and planned to finish the fall working at the SJSU dining commons before attending on-campus classes in the spring in San Francisco. He would walk to the light rail on the other side of Japantown and take it to the Cal-train station near downtown San Jose. From there, he'd take the two-hour ride all the way to the King's street station in San Francisco, walk to a nearby school building and use the school shuttle to go to another building in the Mission District and another near Pier 39. He'd do four, three-hour classes and then make the trip back home.

At the beginning of October 2011, Warren began talking to a co-worker, a red-headed El Salvadorian and invited her to a couple of parties at his townhome in Japantown. When she asked Warren to make her his girlfriend, he told her he was too messed up to be with anyone. So, he stopped talking to her. At that point, Warren had dated a few times but had no interest in forming relationships with any of them. A week after refusing the co-worker from the dining commons, however, another girl would catch Warren's eye and would hold it forever. One day on a Tuesday, while at work at the

SJSU dining commons, Warren left the back-kitchen area to go on break. As he walked around one of the server bars, a white Mexican American student, who was standing in line at the sandwich bar with an Ethiopian roommate and a Nigerian friend, caught Warren's gaze. He froze on her face and they locked eyes. Later, she told Warren that her friends had asked who the guy was that was staring at her, and she told them that she didn't know, but Warren responded he thought she was looking at him first. Warren finished his break and then completed his shift. Over the next day or so, Warren saw her each time he made his rounds to fill the server bars. She passed by with her roommate and friends and would always meet Warren's eyes and smile. He later discovered that she stayed in the Joe West dormitory building attached to the dining commons.

Finally, one day, Warren saw her again waiting in line at the Latin bar with her roommate. He went to fill the salad and yogurt bar, and she met his eyes again as he walked past. When he filled the bar and walked past her back toward the kitchen, he stopped. He turned to her and said he felt he knew her from a social media page. He asked her what her name was. "Willow," she said, beaming brightly. Warren shrugged and decided she wasn't who he thought she was, so he accepted he didn't know her after all. When Warren searched for roommates on the SJSU social media group page, he came across a comment from a student regarding sports. A debate ensued about bandwagons and championship hoppers, and he ceased replying after they compiled a lengthy thread. He thought this girl was Willow. Glad that it wasn't, he walked back into the kitchen. He stopped after taking about three steps and felt he should at least give her his name, too. He walked back to Willow and said, "Hi, I am Warren." He smiled and held out his hand. Willow grinned, shook his hand, and said it was nice to meet him, and he returned to work.

The next day, Warren received a friend request on Facebook from Willow and he quickly accepted it. Within a minute, he sent her a message saying *hello*. She responded immediately and he asked her on a date. She accepted and they planned for the following Monday. A few days before the date, however, on a Friday, Warren and his roommates went bowling on the SJSU campus. Warren invited Willow to come out and bowl at the alley, which was on the lowest level of the student union building. At first, she said she was hanging out with friends, but after Warren and his friends showed up on her floor in one of the common areas, she and her friends agreed to go. As they walked to the student union building from Joe West, it started raining. Although Willow had a white leather jacket on, Warren took off his coat and put it on her anyway. They went bowling, laughed, had fun, and then he walked her back to her dorm. After he dropped off Willow, Warren's roommates praised him for how beautiful she was and encouraged him to keep dating her.

On November 9th, 2011, they went on their first date. Just as Warren once looked up and saw the devil Paul as he came out of his job and stared down at him and his mother before he ran their family to the ground so long ago, Warren now stood at the top stair of his job at the dining commons looking down to the bottom at an angel – Willow. She waited patiently for him with a warm smile. They walked holding hands to a three-story cinema downtown and watched Paranormal Activity Two. It was here they first kissed and Warren asked her to be his girlfriend. She said yes. Afterward, they walked a couple of blocks to La Victoria, a popular Mexican restaurant in San Jose and had dinner. Warren then walked Willow back across campus from San Carlos street to her dorm at Joe West, kissed her goodnight, and then returned to his home in Japantown. They had grown closer as friends ever since.

***

One day, Warren invited Willow over to cook her pasta. She agreed and Warren made so much they prepared to share with other housemates when they returned home. One of Warren's housemates, a curly-headed light-skinned African American from Los Angeles, had a bad habit of getting blackout drunk anytime he partied. That evening, he had been at a neighbor's home drinking relentlessly while his girlfriend remained in his bedroom. When Warren and

Willow finished their supper, his housemate stumbled inside with black rings around his eyes. His Latin girlfriend quickly came down to retrieve him. However, he became resistant to her and pushed her away. He told her to stay away from him and when she persisted in getting close, he grabbed her and threw her into a wall. He then proceeded to sock her repeatedly in the face and head. This was the first time Warren had seen a woman get hit since his mother so many years ago. Warren jumped from his seat beside Willow and intervened. He tried to redirect his housemate, but he got prideful. He threatened to hit Warren if he didn't move out of his way. When Warren held his ground, his housemate reeled a punch and delivered it. Warren countered the attack and took his housemate's head and began driving it into the same wall he had thrown his girlfriend into. They fought their way into the living room, where the housemate tried to swing at Warren again. Warren attempted to counter it with a silly martial art move he knew well and had taught the housemate just days prior, and before he could complete the move, his housemate bit him hard on the inner bicep and gritted his teeth. Warren drove him through a table and into the ground. The fight ended when Warren stood up and realized he had broken his right hand and that his forehead had a long, bleeding cut across it. He was later told his head either went through a corner table as they fell or he was hit in the head with a hookah base. Warren couldn't remember which caused his head to bleed. His lip was also swollen and his inner bicep stung from his housemate's bite. Warren led Willow outside and the police got called. Warren was sent to the hospital to be put into a cast and received antibiotics for his bite mark and cuts. His housemate went to jail. However, the next day, Warren and Willow learned that his girlfriend had bailed him out. After Warren was treated and told he needed to quit smoking cigarettes, which he did, he and Willow returned to his home in Japantown and she took good care of him that week. This was the first time Warren told her he loved her.

He muttered, "I think I l.o.v.e. you," one evening, as she applied ointment to his forehead.

"I think I l.o.v.e. you, too," Willow replied. They had grown closer as lovers ever since.

Chapter IX: The Great Central Valley

In Warren's second year at the Academy of Art University, he began freelancing on film, television, and media production sets. Having begun his freelancing career on an unpaid web series, Warren eventually got referred by many peers and hiring managers into paid gigs. Warren worked on many productions, including sports broadcasting, where he got to meet Steph Curry and the champion Golden State Warriors in Oakland in between their '17 and '18 championships, watched the San Jose Sharks play the LA Kings from their locker room, and worked behind the scenes at the '17 Pac-12 Championship game and Super Bowl 50 when they were hosted at Levi's Stadium. Warren worked all over the San Francisco Bay Area for sports broadcasting, commercials, documentaries, and short films.

He spread his reach into the Great Central Valley, where he worked on a Scott Peterson documentary, Monterey Bay, where he worked on MTV's Catfish, and then down to Los Angeles, where he worked on an Indy film with a murderous storyline. He also got hired at the cinema in downtown San Jose where he and Willow had their first date and later got promoted to assistant manager. Warren, confident in his freelancing career and unable to afford the high tuition at the Academy of Art, discontinued film school and attended De Anza Community College in Cupertino. Warren liked this campus because it was brown and beautiful and because he got to drive by the Apple Headquarters every day, but he struggled to remain focused in class and consistent with his work. Although he attended a screenwriting seminar that his teacher hosted and even joined a film club and sat on the student government council as their representative, Warren felt it best to discontinue his schooling after a year of struggling mentally, financially, and emotionally. He also grew even more distant from the housemate with who he fought. His housemate moved back in after he got bailed out and had fallen out of school. Warren packed up his belongings one day and moved into Willow's new dorm at the Campus Villages Building. After a couple of semesters of living on campus with her, they rented a room together in a big blue house close to the corner of 15th and Julian.

For a week one summer, Willow invited Warren to visit her and her father's side of the family in South Texas. Every summer since her parents divorced, she and her sister made it a tradition to visit him in Brownsville, right on the border of Mexico. Warren landed in Harlingen and Willow picked him up in her dad's Toyota Tundra. The weather was hot and humid, and it rained randomly, to Warren's surprise. Warren liked Willow's dad.

He ran a small but popular tortilla factory on the same block that he and most of his family lived on. They all owned land and had built homes and businesses on them. Willow's Dad rented a condo on South Padre Island for them and her cousins for three days. They loaded up the Tundra and Willow drove everyone to the island. They checked into their condo, went to Schlitterbahn waterpark, ate at Whataburger, and shopped for souvenirs along the island. Warren swam in the Gulf of Mexico and loved the warm water. In comparison to the Atlantic and Pacific Oceans, he told Willow, the gulf water was warm and felt amazing.

At the end of December 2015, Willow received her Bachelor's degree in Sociology with a minor in Justice Studies. Warren couldn't have been any prouder. This inspired him to pursue a degree again. He took her graduation photos and attended her graduation when she walked at the end of spring with her friends. A couple of months later, she received her diploma in December. Warren and Willow decided to take some time away from the Bay Area to take care of her mother for a year. Warren was from Stockton and Fresno, and he was intrigued by the fact that Willow and her family resided in the Modesto area, which sits somewhere in the middle between the two. Although Warren vowed never to move back to the Great Central Valley, in mid of February 2016, they moved to a little country home off Grayson Road. The timing of the move worked out perfectly with Warren's decision to pause freelancing because his other job at the cinema had been faced with high rent from the city and the cinema could no longer afford to sustain itself despite efforts to fundraise and collaborate with vendors. It closed in summer of 2016. Warren was glad it did. He disliked his co-workers most of the time. When he first got hired as a floor staff member, some of the employees were rude when they trained him, gossiped behind his back, and never helped him close. When he worked hard enough to get promoted to assistant manager, he found himself retaliating against those that acted negatively toward him when he was floor staff by being overbearing, controlling, and a micromanager. Anytime employees showed up late, burned popcorn, or hid away in the auditoriums to watch movies when they were supposed to be working, Warren was on them with a write-up. He eventually calmed down when they began to respect him, but he felt he had to become strict to gain fear and, thus, gain respect. Warren quit around the time he and Willow moved and word of the cinema's closure caught up to him while working at his next job. Before Warren quit, however, the housemate, he fought visited the cinema a few times to watch movies and they reconciled. To Warren, he had met worse than this housemate and understood the pain and struggle he was experiencing. He wished him well.

For the year, Warren and Willow lived with her mother. He helped them plant a garden in the backyard. He dug the weeds out of the ground and assembled planter boxes.

Willow's aunt helped by buying plants and her mother helped by having a friend of hers build a deck. When that finished, Warren helped load logs into a tractor for an almond orchard landowner who also owned the land that Willow's mother lived on. He also applied to work part-time at a Fairfield Inn and Suites in Turlock. After three months of working there, he got employee of the month appreciation, and then a few months after that, he got promoted to full-time. Soon, however, probably because of his success, Warren didn't like his co-workers there either. During his first two weeks of working at the hotel, two other staff members, a female Sikh Pakistani and a male, blue-eyed white atheist, thought it wise to ask Warren what his religion was. Warren made the mistake of discussing the topic, but he told them he was a Christian. Ever since, Warren felt rude and disrespectful comments. The female co-worker would hover, micromanage, and then gossip nonstop behind Warren's back. While in a meeting, the male co-worker, who became a front desk manager, tried to embarrass Warren in front of everyone by trying to make him look incompetent when he asked a question. Warren, tired of the attitudes of his fellow co-workers, argued with the front desk manager in front of everyone at the meeting.

Shortly afterward, the hotel's general manager was fired for impregnating his head of housekeeping and then replaced by the front desk manager, who hired Warren. Then, a sales manager position became available and it was all the talk and buzz around the property. Warren's co-workers, who were mainly women, wanted to apply for the position, but due to some reason, tensions arose and gossip spiked toward Warren. He felt himself becoming public enemy number one. He figured it was because people saw him as a threat to their promotion. When his co-worker's attitudes began to affect him, Warren responded with some of his own. But, this only made matters worse as one-sided complaints were being made against him. Warren had to meet with the new general manager and explain himself. He told her the issues began when he told people his religion when he started, and ever since, the harassment had been nonstop.

A day later, the female Sikh Pakistani co-worker who led in the harassment was terminated. Warren didn't stick around long enough to see what would happen to the male co-worker because he had already been long affected by his treatment since he started at the hotel. A disgruntled, rude, and arrogant customer walked in one day, asked for a room, and when Warren told him they were full, the customer acted belligerent. Warren gave the man an annoyed, disgruntled look, and the man raised a complaint to his manager, saying Warren was threatening him. Warren was called into the office to explain himself, but wasn't reprimanded.

The next day, he quit anyway. A position became available in Atlanta, Georgia, that intrigued Warren. It was an associate producer job for a well-established media production company that had an Emmy award-winning show. A distant cousin was going to help him to get the position as she was helping with the hiring process, held the position herself, and was looking for her replacement. However, at the end of winter in 2016, Warren found he did not get the position and it was the first time he realized that he needed a college degree if he was going to ever be competitive in the hiring process, get the job, and make substantial, consistent money so he can attain a better life for him and Willow. He paused media production freelancing, applied for Merced College, and in June of 2017, he and Willow moved again. However, about a month before they moved, Warren convinced Willow to take a trip with him back to San Jose. They met up with a childhood friend of Willow's and went on a hike on Communications Hill. This hill was less than a mile from the Catholic church where Willow's parents had gotten married long ago. Warren had only told her friend at the time, but while he was in Santa Cruz working on the show, The Drone Racing League, he had taken a stroll along the beach after his shift ended and came across drone flyers. He befriended them and they let him fly one. He took their contact information and a week later asked one of them to come to San Jose to film his proposal to Willow. The flyer agreed and offered to do it without charge. The flyer met Warren and the two ladies at

Communications Hill and recorded themselves as they climbed it. Warren told Willow that his friend was testing out the features of the drone.

When they got to the top of the hill, Warren pulled out the ring and proposed while the drone continued to record and Willow exclaimed yes. The flyer created a short film of the recording and they believed they were one of the first couples to propose that way because public drone flying had just become a thing a few years prior.

They moved into a house in North Merced and Warren started volunteering at the county food bank and at a youth grieving nonprofit over the summer until school at Merced College could start in the fall. Willow got a job as a social worker aide at the Merced County Human Services Agency before transferring to Behavioral Health and Recovery Services as a Mental Health Worker. When school started in the fall for Warren, he took on 16-plus units to finish in a two-year time frame. After achieving straight A-s in his first semester, he decided to get involved in extracurricular activities. While sitting in the Lesher building one day, waiting for his name to get called to see an academic advisor, two African American female school counselors approached him and asked if he wanted to join a club. When he asked what club, they told him it was the Black Student Union and they were searching for people to fill some vacant positions. Warren attended a meeting and agreed to be their student council representative. After two weeks, the president of the club informed the advisors she couldn't do the position anymore and they called Warren. They told him it was discussed by the rest of the club and decided to make him their next president. Warren was flattered to have been preselected and accepted the position.

Chapter X: Merced

Warren designed the Black Student Union's logo, helped everyone decide what attire they were going to purchase, and had their logo embroidered into it. He then tweaked the constitution and bylaws to protect himself as the president of the club. Warren knew people and he felt all the power resided in the constitution. He had looked it over and felt it was too weak and asked to amend it. The club advisors agreed and approved the changes.

Everything changed when the club became official after winter break and Warren was, in a sense, given the keys to lead it. An unruly black student by the name of Corinthia tried to join the club, but the advisors despised her. They told Warren not to let her into the club. Warren felt this was against the club's goals and purpose and encouraged her to join. This angered his club's advisors and board members, and they held a meeting off-campus. When Warren arrived, he was surprised to find that it was an ambush. They had set the meeting up to remove him from his position as president of the Black Student Union.

Before this meeting began, Warren had prayed. He knew something was up and didn't want to deal with the stress and anxiety of it. So, he asked God for help. Before Warren arrived at the meeting, he emailed everyone the new constitution and bylaws they approved. When everyone arrived for the meeting, they knew he meant business. His advisors barely looked at him when they walked into the meeting house and waited for the debate. Warren let everyone speak their peace first. They felt he didn't listen to their advice and requests.

Warren reminded him he was well within his power to do what he did and for them to try and remove him from his position in the way they tried was illegal and unethical. He told them to give him another chance to make things right, and they agreed to let him remain and ended the meeting.

However, matters only got worse as the next two months went by when Corinthia kept trying to get into the club and Warren let her. The advisors quit and the board disbanded. Then, Warren began to regret every decision he had made up to that point as Corinthia became the very monster he was warned to be. She turned most of the club against Warren, openly argued with him in front of everyone in every meeting, gossiped behind his back, and conspired to remove him from his position. Warren couldn't believe the mess he had let unfold. He had joined this club to try and do something for his people, but this was the appreciation and treatment he got. He let Corinthia have her way and control every event and thing the club did. Warren knew she aspired to be the next student body president of the school and had been planning to run for the student government elections at the end of the spring semester. Warren had no intention of ever running, but when Corinthia insulted him at an event and embarrassed him in front of everyone, he erupted in anger, yelled at her in the quad, and then put the word out that he would be her running mate in the upcoming student government elections. Warren had been taking anxiety medication for a brief period around this time and he had ingested a pill without the required water amount shortly before this heated argument. After Warren drove off and just as he got to his house, he felt the pill dissolve and burn his insides. He figured his argument with Corinthia accelerated its properties, and for the first time in his life, he felt his anger turned on him.

After he recovered, he ceased taking the medication. It was Corinthia's third year running for the student body president position and he refused to let her get it. There was a third running mate, a student named Pablo, but when he found out Warren was going to run against Corinthia, he stepped down to advise him instead. When the campaign event began in May 2018, Warren marketed himself nobly and respectfully while Corinthia went into the classrooms and meeting halls to announce all the negative aspects she perceived of Warren. She barely knew Warren, as he was new in the town and campus, so he couldn't figure out where she was getting his information. Anyhow, she insulted and slandered him everywhere she went. When word got back to Warren, even from teachers, that she was spreading ill-word about him to half the campus, he lost motivation and felt he'd lose the campaign, but his supporters kept encouraging him to keep trying and that people like her wouldn't win. Warren stuck to his campaign strategy of being welcoming, approachable, respectable, and honest. When the votes were counted, Warren had 50% of the vote, Corinthia had 42%, and 8% of the votes were neutral. He had beaten Corinthia and was the new student body president of Merced College.

Over the summer, Warren trained for the pro bono position, becoming familiar with state and federal laws, education codes, administrative policies and procedures, Robert's Rules of Order, and the Brown Act. He also signed up for American Government and Political Science classes. He filled the remaining seats on the executive board of the student organization and the vacant senatorial positions and then set forth a platform that his cabinet and administration could support. He had a course load of 16-plus units, was the associated student body president, had gotten re-elected president of the Black Student Union, and then got hired on-campus as an embedded peer mentor for writing and literacy.

While Warren became distracted by his full course load, Pablo, the student government clerk who stepped aside to let Warren run against Corinthia, got bored. His role was in graphic designing and anything in leadership. Not only was this clerk a part-time student, but he was also getting paid for his role in student government. He had a lot of time on his hands to undermine anything Warren said or did. Warren had heard rumors of this clerk before he began and how he liked to make power moves and provide rude customer service. He even butted heads with the former student body president.

Warren had been warned. He knew if he was going to run a positive administration built on good service and trust, then this clerk's sort of behavior was going to have to stay away, but Warren met with him anyway to find common ground and see what they could accomplish together. They ended their meeting and Warren thought they'd be fine going forward, but one day, as he approached the office during business hours, he saw that it was dark inside. When he unlocked the door and stepped in, he saw the clerk sitting in the dark with a few of his friends, gossiping. Warren held a meeting later in the month to go over ground rules, goals, and the plan for the rest of the academic year. Objectives were agreed upon and everyone parted to go about their duties. As the semester progressed, Warren came to find that Pablo tested and undermined him any chance he got. Not only did he persist in influencing those Warren recruited into the organization, but anytime they were at an event or in public, Pablo would try to take control of the events and embarrass him in front of others. He would also be rude, disrespectful, and persist in sabotaging anything Warren said or did. Anytime tasks were given, or anything was set forth in the motion, Warren would wait until the document upon which it was written would disappear and would expect there to be errors and hiccups in the student council meetings and in follow-up conversations. By the middle of Warren's academic year as a student body president, roughly half of Warren's cabinet seemed indifferent to him or, at the very least, distracted from the mission and vision they all agreed upon and adopted. Anything he said wrong, did, or didn't do was talked about negatively, but anytime he did anything that was successful, no one said anything. He felt that presidency, like everything else in the past, had struggled because someone else couldn't stand to see him succeed. Still, Warren got to sit in a room with governor-elect Gavin Newsom, Mayor Mike Murphy, and all of Merced College's and the city's leadership in one room at the campus Library. There is a picture of Warren with them. He was standing in the middle of the groundbreaking event of the new Agricultural-IT building. There was another picture of Warren standing with the governor, assemblyman Adam Gray, and an agricultural honor roll student.

In the winter of 2018, after the Camp Fire blew up Paradise, California, Warren put together a relief effort through the college for his student government team to launch and see through. He campaigned and gathered donations campus-wide, reserved two vans, and when he went to load them up, no one in his team helped. Instead, some members tried to distract him by signing papers he had to take two looks at because he realized it was something he did not want to sign. Pablo even tried to say something negative about the relief effort in terms of only doing it for publicity. Warren ignored them and when the two volunteers from outside of the student organization arrived, one of the faculty members from the Merced campus and one a student from the Los Banos campus, boarded the vans and drove to Butte County, which is North of Sacramento. They dropped off the donations at an encampment with success and returned to Merced in a matter of a few hours.

***

Earlier that year, in August, before drama escalated within his presidency and right after Warren had completed his student government summer training, he received a Facebook message from someone claiming to be his older sister. Warren had only ever known two siblings, an older sister, and a brother before they got split up after their mother's death. When Summer died, Warren was sent to Fresno while his half-sister, who was thought to be the oldest of Summer's children at the time, remained in Stockton with her grandmother and their half-brother was sent to live with his dad in Las Vegas. Ever since the three siblings hardly remained in contact. As they would get older, contact would slowly but surely improve. However, it fragmented. Warren hadn't checked his Facebook messages in about a month. He noticed he had an unread one. Before he even opened the message, the woman in the profile picture immediately reminded him of his mother. If anything, he thought it could have been a sister of hers, but when he opened the message, which was about three weeks old, the lady said that she was his sister and that she found him through their mother's Coroner's report. In the report, she read that Summer was having chest pains in the days leading up to her death, and when she passed away, she was survived by three kids. That information, combined with using social media, enabled her to locate them easily. When Warren confirmed who he was, she explained that Summer had three children with her first husband, the Navy Sailor, who brought her back to the United States after the Vietnam War. They had two sons and a girl. She told Warren that when her dad came home one day, Summer was gone and nowhere to be found. She had abandoned her children, all under the age of six, and left no note. They would grow up and experience life in Portsmouth, Virginia, and have children of their own and then grandchildren. Warren never knew he had about 20 nieces and nephews. Up to this point, Warren had known nothing of Summer's past. Even when Warren spoke to Dominic, he said she was good at keeping her past in the dark and never spoke about it. Warren had given up and accepted the fact that his mother was the best secret keeper he had ever known.

Dominic had gotten out of prison two years before

Warren enlisted in the military. While Warren was living in Stockton with Benjamin, after he returned from his training in North Carolina and before he moved to San Jose, he spoke with and visited Dominic in Vallejo. Dominic worked at a recycling plant in American Canyon, lived in a townhouse off Sacramento street in Vallejo, and was engaged to a white woman ten years older than him. Warren spent the night a couple of times and would eventually introduce Willow to them when they lived in San Jose. He'd play basketball, go to the gym, and even watch a movie at a local cinema with Dominic and his fiancé. Warren and Dominic would grow distant when Warren began to struggle in San Jose and this worsened as he moved to Merced. Through his conversations with Dominic, he came to realize that he didn't need a Dad. He had outgrown and gone far in life without one and felt that he truly was better off without him, even as friends. Warren believed his relationship deterioration with Dominic began when he asked him questions about Summer and didn't get any answers. Instead, he found out Dominic had gotten Summer on drugs, namely cocaine, in the year leading up to his conception and birth and that she had been addicted ever since. This, on top of many other things, in combination with the ups and downs Warren was experiencing at the time, led him to feel that Dominic was still a child, and he, therefore, ceased speaking to him.

Warren later found out, in the middle of his student presidency and after he had just discovered he had long-lost siblings, that Dominic was homeless. Right before Thanksgiving Day in 2018, Dominic had gotten into odds with his fiancé. Tensions had been boiling for some time since he had lost his job and his townhome and then became homeless. While his former fiancé had social security benefits that enabled her to live in a well-protected living community after eviction, however, Dominic did not. He was an unemployed former felon and was regulated to the streets of Vallejo. When this happened, his fiancé began to cheat and Dominic caught her in the middle of the act one evening. He never trusted her again and when she asked him to move in, he chose to be homeless instead and called off whatever wedding they would have had. This was when he began to use drugs again, namely methamphetamines. Warren remembered when he had looked over the autopsy report that his long-lost half-sister sent him. It revealed the same drug was in Summer's system at the time she died. Warren reasoned that it was Dominic who got Summer on cocaine and then Paul who got her on meth. He then reasoned that his mother probably allowed both into her system as some sort of self-reckoning punishment for what she allowed to happen to her family. Warren believed his mother had been punishing herself, even with Paul's abuse for those last two years of her life, because she felt she deserved it.

While attending Merced College, Warren got wind of a sweeping movement to improve mental health awareness nationwide. His organization would collaborate with nonprofit and government agencies who would come out to campus to the table and market their services, as well as hand out freebies such as t-shirts, buttons, and pens. Warren knew he struggled with some underlying issues through most of his teenage years and young adult life because of what had happened to him throughout his childhood, but he didn't know most of his social issues were the result of not having dealt with these problems at all. Then, in October of 2018, while going to school full-time, doing student leadership and tutoring, as well as working the front desk at a hotel in South Merced, Warren's eye got infected. He later attributed it to stress and working in unsanitary working conditions, but it worsened over the next two days before he finally saw a doctor who quickly referred him to an eye specialist. Warren didn't take the prescribed eye drops on time and with the proper dosage before he fell asleep that night. In the middle of the night, he awoke in pain from his eye-searing. He flicked on the bathroom light and was shocked to see that one of his eyes had a grey spot covering the lens. As he was about to panic into oblivion, Warren felt an overwhelmingly good feeling in his heart that assured him that he would be okay. The feeling made Warren confident he would recover from this pain and blindness. So, Warren chose the good reassuring feeling over fear and panic and remained calm.

The eye specialist, a young woman, and the daughter of the owner of the practice diagnosed Warren with severe iritis. She said his pupil had swollen and attached to his lens and he would require steroid drops in the eye every morning before school for the next month or two. Warren couldn't believe it. After all he'd been through in life, he now had temporary blindness. The specialist told him he may never see the same in it and said if she didn't use steroids, then the inflammation would never break and his blurred vision and the excruciating pain he'd been experiencing would become permanent. He refused to endure such a thing and every day for a month before class and his shift at the student government office, he would have to go and sit under her hand for steroid droplets, and blinding light. Of all aspects of the healing process that hurt the most was the light that she beamed into his eye. Each time, his inflamed eye would feel weak under the strength of the light and resort to flooding out tears. By the time Warren finished his rehabilitation, he had joked that he couldn't cry out of the eye anymore, but he healed, and when the specialist examined him and then when he went and got a second opinion, he was told that his vision was better in the eye than before. Warren thanked God.

Chapter XI: God

Over the course of November and into December, after healing from his ailment, stress resumed in Warren. He had flooded his plate with too many obligations and was losing sight and control of it all. Having a high unit course load, student involvement, two jobs, and then the increasing drama in his social life, Warren felt he had overexerted and exhausted his energy. For the past fourteen years, he has been facing trouble sleeping due to many reasons, one of them being sleep paralysis. In his first event, he experienced what felt like an airplane engine being lowered on him while he lay frozen in the dark. Another similar event that stood out above the rest was when he felt a helicopter propeller, fully powered on, also being lowered on him in the dark. The rest of the events Warren experienced over that fourteen-year time frame was similar in theme and their frequency and strength depended solely on what he was going and feeling through at that time in his life. Each time in sleep paralysis, he was frozen in darkness and fully conscious.

The last event, one that seemed to evolve each night for three nights that December, had manifested into something Warren had yet to experience in any of his sleep paralysis episodes and it was enough to scare him into running back to church. The first night was more of a nightmare. He could move around in the dark, but he knew someone had just broken into the house downstairs. He stood at his bedroom door in the dark, waiting for whoever it was to get to him upstairs. Unsure of what to do in the dream, Warren asked God for help. That was when he woke up and told Willow. On the second night, Warren went into sleep paralysis as he tried to descend into slumber. The room was pitch dark and his body froze again. To his surprise, and unlike any other episode before, Warren felt a child climb into bed with him in the dark from where his feet lay. He assumed it was a demon. It crawled up his legs and then sat on Warren's chest, making it hard for him to breathe. He could feel his body depressing into the mattress from the weight of it and then, it rang a bell in Warren's ear for what felt like four seconds. As Warren's fear spiked, that's when it happened. From his heart, he exclaimed, "Christ, save me!"

As if someone flipped on a switch, lightly pouring into the room from outside. It felt as if it was never dark and that the darkness had been nothing but a figment of Warren's imagination. Outside his bedroom window, as he continued to lie on his bed, he felt like a new dream. Warren could see what looked like three large white seagulls circling above. Suddenly, they swirled down to Warren and swooped him upward before he could blink. He felt as if his soul had been lifted out of his body and he was getting taken upwards on a journey with big white birds which continued to swirl around him. They lifted Warren out of bed and into a galactic funnel cloud. He could see stars through the smoke. Warren thought he was traveling up through a tornado to the heavens. At the top of the funnel, he could see white light, dark space, and then a metallic face peering down at him. The face looked as if it was made of silvery tungsten. It smiled at Warren and he smiled back. Then, as if gravity kicked back on, Warren free fell through the funnel and back into his room, landing on the floor. Warren got up, ran downstairs and was surprised to see that the rear sliding door was ajar. It made him think of the first dream he had the night prior when he heard it open and waited for the intruder to come upstairs. Warren woke up and his back felt sore. He told Willow.

Later that day, Warren paid a visit to a youth pastor at a nearby church called Gateway. Warren had started going to this church on and off since he and Willow moved to Merced. He then attended the college classes the youth pastor would host weekly on the church campus. When he began experiencing stress and sleep paralysis, he wanted answers. Warren utilized the pastor for Christian counseling services. He asked Warren to catch him up and he told him his story about his recent experiences with sleep paralysis. The pastor looked at books and into his own theologian knowledge and connected the events to something traumatic that may have happened in Warren's early life. Warren accepted this and looked to go about his days in peace, forgiveness, and in harmony. However, on that night, the third night, Warren had another sleep paralysis event and when he tried to call out to Christ for help again, nothing happened. His tormentor locked him into his frozen state and the episode played out as usual.

The next day, Warren told the pastor and after some deliberation, they concluded that calling Christ only truly worked if it was said from the heart. So, they planned to be prepared for the next event.

That night, Warren slipped into another episode. When he felt the darkness closing in and his tormentor gaining in, he began chanting Christ's name from within. At first, he could feel its powerful effects working as if it was an invisible force field, but as soon as he started saying it with his mind, the force field deteriorated and the dark force broke through and bound him to the remainder of the episode. Warren didn't see the pastor the next day and fell into another episode that night. This time, Warren was fed up, annoyed, and prepared. He was going to use his short temper and flip his switch on this demon. He wanted this thing to leave him alone and he knew he was stronger than this. He refused to be fucked with any longer. When Warren felt the negative energy and his tormentor closing in, he flipped on his willpower. From his heart, he harnessed what belief, love, and spiritual power he had in Christ and let it flow out as if it was his own power to use. Warren remembered what the pastor told him, "Your name is written in heaven."

It worked as if Warren's spirit had turned into a force field that was channeled by a supernatural or divine power. It projected outward in an instant and repelled the incoming tormentor. Warren could feel the energy radiating from his body, working in his favor. The darkness and his tormentor were vanquished and Warren woke from his nightmare. This was the last time he experienced sleep paralysis. When Warren told the youth pastor, he was thrilled. He was so excited he told Warren that if it did come back, then he was confident Warren could use his name in Heaven to call out the demon's name, stop it dead in its tracks, and make it obey him. The youth pastor reminded Warren that although he isn't more powerful than the demon and the other dark forces we can't see, he has authority over it. Warren joked he hoped the demon never came back so he wouldn't have to use it.

***

Over the course of winter break that year, Warren continued to see the youth pastor for follow-up sessions. The pastor had been effective in helping Warren back onto his spiritual journey, getting to know God better, and overcoming something that had plagued him most of his life. On the last day Warren met him, the pastor told him he wanted to further help his situation by making sure he corrected everything in his life that possibly attracted such level of darkness. Warren knew his temper, impatience, and lack of forgiveness were a problem, but he wasn't too sure what other issue there could be especially considering he had just defeated his night terrors with belief.

"I know you're going to say God would never tell me to divorce my wife, but," the youth Pastor started. "You are a Christian and your fiancé is a Catholic."

"What do you mean, Pastor?" Warren asked. He had been wondering if the pastor would marry them.

"A Christian should marry a Christian," the pastor said, treading softly. "So that in matrimony, they can remain aligned in mind, body, spirit, as well as in the faith."

The pastor then told Warren that he was picky with who he would marry as clergy and that he doesn't marry just anyone. He then said that if Warren wanted to marry her, then they would need to split up first. Warren didn't understand. He felt Willow was a gift from God and now this pastor wanted to risk ending their relationship before it could be made to last forever. Warren practically fell into tears when he heard this and tried to reason with the youth pastor, but with the pastor having a strong theologian background and history in the Baptist church and having brought his talents to a community church, there was no swaying his judgment. Warren went home, told Willow what the pastor told him and together, they felt disrespected. Willow fell into tears. They never returned to that church.

***

Warren married Willow in March of 2019. A few months later, Willow's mother had been planning a family reunion in the Phoenix and Las Vegas areas earlier that year and the couple saw this as an opportunity to get hitched. Up to that point, they hadn't planned their wedding and were waiting until Warren graduated from college. Willow told her parents they were going to elope in Las Vegas and then her mother coordinated for the family reunion to take place there so they could have a decent small wedding instead. Willow's father planned to fly out from Texas with his new wife and Warren, in the month leading up to the wedding, decided to find Dominic, who was still homeless on the streets of Vallejo.

He and Willow had to take two trips to Vallejo to find and retrieve Dominic. On the first trip, Warren entered the building where his father's former fiancé lived. He managed to bypass the security entry when someone exited. He had visited there before when Dominic lived there briefly years in the past and didn't remember which apartment was hers. He reached an upper floor, about the same eye level he had remembered from her kitchen view and matched it with the current view he had from a hallway window. He then adjusted his position to the eye frame he remembered and landed at a unit that had a hallway light out next to it. It turned on with Warren's motion. When Warren knocked on

98

the door, he paused and waited. He was surprised when Dominic's former fiancé answered. She looked the same as before; white, elderly, and smelled of cigarettes. She welcomed him in and he kindly asked about whereabouts of Dominic. She said the last time she saw Dominic, they had an argument and he never came back. Warren asked where he could have set up camp and she gave him a couple of pointers. He got into the car where Willow was waiting. Together they drove around downtown, the waterfront, library and circled a grocery outlet countless times trying to find him. Warren even approached a few homeless people and encampments to inquire if he was there. When it got too dark and started to rain, they returned home to Merced.

On the second trip, during the week leading up to the wedding, Warren got a call from Dominic's former fiancé. She said she ran into Dominic while at the grocery outlet and told him Warren was looking for him and that he was getting married. She said Dominic agreed to go with her to get cleaned up and prepared. When Warren and Willow drove up to Vallejo to pick him up two days before the wedding, it was as if Dominic had a different look in his eye. He looked tired and exhausted but didn't appear homeless. This was the first time he had seen Dominic in two years. Warren wondered if he was high but didn't bother to inquire. He had cleaned up well. The four of them went out to dinner at a Chinese buffet restaurant and it was here that Dominic asked

Warren out of nowhere and in front of Willow, "So, why are you getting married? I never got married." Warren didn't say anything right away and Willow excused herself to fill a void on her plate at the buffet. "Because it's the right thing to do," Warren replied, in the deep American voice he had inherited from Dominic. "When are you two getting married? How did that work out?" Dominic smiled and muttered a joke about the answer to his former fiancé as she nervously ate before he returned to his own dinner. Warren excused himself to refill his plate and returned to the table with Willow. The dinner was going well after that, with hardly anyone exchanging words until Dominic went on a sudden tirade about then President Donald Trump's Space Wars plan. He was thrilled about the idea and began talking in such enthusiasm that a man eating with his wife at a table beside them excused himself from his table to refill his plate. Warren redirected Dominic to another topic of discussion and when they finished eating, they retrieved what few belongings Dominic had for the trip and traveled to Merced.

They spent one night in Merced, and the next day, Willow's mother, sister and brother retrieved her and went ahead to Las Vegas to meet her father, who had flown in from Texas. Warren had called his cousin, who was the son of Aunt Tania, who defended his actions when he left them that night, to be his best man. Willow's sister would serve as her maid-of-honor. The cousin drove down from

Sacramento, picked up Warren and Dominic, and followed the others to Vegas. Warren and Willow filed for their marriage license the night they arrived in the city and the next day, at the Fremont Wedding Chapel in the Neonopolis, which is a mile from the cemetery where Grandma Peace and Madea are buried, they got married. Warren remembered it raining that evening and there being a full moon present as they waited for their event to begin. Willow told him these were the good signs.

Warren's Aunt Sheryl, who was the only daughter born to his grandfather, Samuel Peace, also attended the wedding. He had also invited Aunt Rhonda after a period of forgiveness, but due to her living in New York and having multiple health issues, she couldn't make it. Warren heard stories of his Aunt Sheryl before he even lived with Aunt Rhonda. Before moving back to Las Vegas in the early 80s, Sheryl terrorized Rhonda in some of the most horrendous ways. Although Sheryl loved and cared for Warren, she abused Rhonda throughout her childhood and then Rhonda would later abuse Warren in his. Sheryl threw a wedding reception barbecue at one of Grandma Peace's sister's house and invited members from the rest of the family. All members present were descendants of the white man who fathered Madea. Madea's mother had other children from her marriage to Mr. Nunn, but Madea was the only one born to a white man and most of her descendants carry a lighter complexion than her siblings'. The majority of Madea's descendants had remained in the Las Vegas, Yuma, and Phoenix areas throughout the mid-to-late 1900s, except for the Peace family, who migrated to Stockton around 1980. They had crammed into a small blue house at the end of Odell avenue on the most Southern tip of Stockton, where Madea's mother lived with a daughter. Almost ten years later, Warren would be born at the San Joaquin General Hospital, less than three miles away. When he had worked odd jobs before he moved to San Jose and met Willow, one of them was as a security guard at the Food 4 Less in the Weston Ranch community, which was across the I- 5 freeway from this house and less than five minutes from the hospital. Stockton will always be Warren's home.

Warren and Willow spent the first two days after their wedding at the Excalibur Hotel and then the rest of the week at the Santa Fe Hotel and Casino with family. They wouldn't go on their honeymoon until three years later. They took a trip to Honolulu, Hawaii, the closest Warren has gotten to his mother's native land, the Philippines. Before Warren brought Dominic to Vegas, he had planned to move him in with Aunt Sheryl so he didn't have to go back to the streets of Vallejo, a homeless man. She agreed to get Dominic back onto his feet and Warren thanked her. Warren bid his farewell to Dominic and left him with his aunt. When their week finished, he and Willow returned home to Merced.

Chapter XII: War and Peace

Warren returned to campus to his full course load. With it being his last semester before transferring colleges and into the upper division, Warren planned to coast out the rest of his obligations with minimal stress. However, he had two pending tasks to see through. Before winter break started the previous semester, he had met the vice president of student services for the school and initiated two motions that he knew would take some time to manifest. The first task Warren had set in motion was the establishment of a paid student events coordinator position. He had convinced the student council the position was needed due to the increase of failed administrative processes and follow-through on discussed plans and events. The motion was passed and Warren waited for the hiring process. In a nutshell, this position would replace the roles of the clerks. He figured that by phasing out or getting rid of the clerks who he felt had manipulated his term, then those who followed or were influenced by them would return to him in loyalty or leave altogether. He was fine with either choice. Warren loved the idea when the vice president of student services pitched it to him and he figured it was the best way to phase out the office clerks he had quickly lost confidence and trust in. When the time came after winter break, Warren was put on the hiring committee for the position and got to screen the candidates.

The second task Warren set in motion before the winter break started was Plan B in case Plan A didn't work to phase out the clerks and still, he'd hope both would play out successfully. When Warren met with the vice president of student services and informed him of the subversive and social bullying-type behavior, he had been experiencing since he took his position, as well as the neglectful oversight of their advisor. They then together agreed that Pablo would be best placed somewhere else. They decided, when the time was right, to move Pablo down the hall from the office to another program. However, this agreement was made with the understanding that Pablo would return to the office once mediation took place and once all issues were sorted out. Warren didn't care. He figured by the time Pablo came back, he would be transferred to the upper division and wouldn't have to see or deal with him any longer. He also had no interest in mediation. Warren wanted to hate Pablo freely and for people to leave him alone about it. When Warren returned from his wedding in late March of 2019, he waited patiently for Pablo to annoy him or get under his skin. Surely enough, within the very first week of Warren's return, he approached Pablo with a task and even wrote it down on a post-it note for him. Pablo grumpily said he'd do it, but when Warren came into the office later in the day, he saw that he was gone and had passed the task onto someone else. It was a classic move Pablo made any time Warren tried to play leader. He would act as if he didn't need to listen or do anything Warren asked despite the fact he was a paid clerk and graphic designer, whereas Warren was only a volunteer. When Warren realized Pablo had evaded another task, he had enough. He met with the vice president of student services that day and told him Pablo needed to go immediately. Within an hour, after Pablo returned from wherever he had disappeared for, the organization advisor entered and met with him privately. Warren went into his own office and closed the door while he waited for the news to break. Within a minute, Pablo knocked on his door. Warren allowed him to enter and he did so with his head down, eyes to the floor. He sat at the chair beside Warren's desk and gently made his appeal. He said he wasn't sure where things went wrong, but he felt that the sudden move was a personal attack on him. Warren didn't say anything. He just sat in silence. When Pablo tried to persuade Warren to change his mind, Warren replied, "The space is best for both of us, but as of now, the best thing for this organization is for you to move down the hallway."

Nothing else was said between them. Pablo got up and left to go appeal to someone else in the administration. Warren, in the meantime, called IT and a kind gentleman came over within five minutes. Warren asked the man to move Pablo's graphic designing computer and workstation out of his former office. The IT specialist did and moved them to the front door. Pablo returned to the office to gather his belongings and saw his moved workstation and finally understood just how Warren truly felt about him. Warren wanted him out and did not care about his feelings. He never got the same treatment from Pablo and now wanted him out of his life. Pablo moved down the hall and this further divided Warren's cabinet and executive board. When people began to speak their minds to Warren about his decision, he ignored them and offered for them to resign if they didn't like it. Then, in a student council meeting, Warren made sure a motion was put on the agenda to vote for the suspension of the funding that paid the clerks' wages. He didn't care about his presidency anymore nor his administration. He even wanted to resign but didn't want to give his so-called political rivals the satisfaction of removing him as the first African American student body president of a Hispanic-serving institution. Warren wanted it all to burn.

Then, one day in April, about two weeks after Pablo's removal from office, a Latina vice-president who Warren appointed at the beginning of his term decided to poke and provoke Warren, which set forth the fire that he needed to expose his unethical organization. The girl had grown close to Pablo and even gave into his politicking influence despite Warren's attempts to forewarn her and thwart his attempts. Warren gave up and let her get close to the person whom he felt she resembled in appearance. Warren would come to view all her attention-seeking ways as betrayal and a distraction to the purpose and mission of the student government organization. When they grew at odds, Warren began to neglect and ignore her. She then began to cast open insults at him in the quad and disrupt him mid-speech in student council meetings. Then, when Pablo was around, she'd purposefully parade their relationship to Warren even after he tried to get her to remain on his side. He gave up on her and, in one student council meeting, asked her to quit. She refused, and when Pablo got kicked out, she entered the office and began openly and sublimely talking smack about Warren being with him nearby. Warren, already annoyed and refusing to hear another word from her, got up from his seat and walked out of the office.

For some reason, she decided to follow him out the door, still provoking him with her speech. When Warren realized the girl was following him, he stopped immediately, turned around, and walked straight past her back into the office to get away. For whatever reason, she perceived this as threatening and walked to human resources in the administration building and reported Warren as having harassed and threatened her. Warren had gone to class and when he returned, the newly-hired student services coordinator, the one he helped hire, stopped him before he could unlock the door to his office. She told him that due to what happened earlier, he was not allowed in the office.

Warren couldn't believe what she was telling him and in the manner and tone in which she was doing it. Warren already didn't like this lady because before she even applied for the position, he had known of her to be close to Pablo in event collaboration. When Warren saw that she made it to the top three candidates of the hiring process, he knew she'd get it and bring Pablo back to the office eventually. So, when she stopped him at his office door to tell him he couldn't go in and that he had to wait for an investigation to be completed, he was appalled. He didn't know what an investigation was needed for. Warren didn't argue, he left the office and focused on class.

When the investigation commenced, Warren was called into the administration building once to give his account of what happened. He told the investigator everything he knew to be true of the drama in the office and what factually took place regarding the harassment claim and left it at that. The investigator informed him of the process that would play out and that he still needed to interview witnesses and others in the organization. He then asked Warren around twenty questions about things that may have or didn't happen over the course of his term and Warren was shocked to find that most of what he was getting asked had been misconstrued or told in a way to benefit the agenda of whoever it was saying it. Warren would later find out that Pablo sat in on one of the investigative interviews and told the investigator things that would later make it back to Warren and confirm to him that he truly was a jealous asshole. Pablo told the investigator that Warren, at one point, sat in his office with the door closed to talk to the treasurer of the organization, whom Warren appointed. Not only was the conversation professional and appropriate, but when they walked out, Pablo was standing in the corner of the outer office with an envious look in his eye anyway. Warren could never understand why Pablo was always lurking around and watching him out of the corner of his eye or anytime he had his back to him. And anytime Warren wanted to talk to anyone in his cabinet, he had to make sure Pablo wasn't around. It all made sense to Warren now; Pablo wanted to be him or, at the very least, see to it that Warren never outshined him or succeeded in any of his goals.

When Warren discovered, through the questions that were being asked, what people had said of him in their interviews, he decided to tell everything that had happened since he got elected. He figured if anyone was going to hear the story of what he went through since he began his fall semester, then it was going to be this investigator who would later pass the findings all the way up to the vice president of student services, the director of human resources, and even the superintendent of the campus. Warren wanted the truth out. So, he told the investigator everything from his perspective that led up to him being accused of harassment and barred from his own office He started with Pablo stepping aside to let him run against Corinthia, then how Pablo and his fellow clerk would openly and behind his back undermine everything he did and how they were subversive to nearly every aspect of his campaign platform, how they influenced his cabinet and basically turned them against him, and how, when he had enough of their politicking and games, he decided to drop a metaphorical hammer on their ways. Warren explained that was when Pablo got kicked out and then his buddy, Warren's own vice president, provoked him shortly afterward and when he tried to flee from her, she twisted the story and accused him of what he currently stood being accused of. The investigator typed everything quickly into his laptop, never breaking eye contact with Warren. When he finished his questions and notes, he dismissed Warren.

***

Warren walked out of the administration building after his interview and saw a recruiting table for Fresno Pacific University, the Merced Campus. He knew the main campus was less than two miles from the Maple Grove apartment complex where he lived with Grandma Peace nearly twenty years earlier and Balderas Elementary school, where he had attended when he and George Jr. were called in to speak with a social worker. Warren approached the table and the Sunbird recruiters welcomed him warmly. He read through the pamphlets, asked questions, and then they ushered him into the first floor of the Lesher Building and ran him through a quick admissions process. They accepted him on the spot and he added the school to his list of transfer options. This was around the time he encouraged and convinced his most trusted friend at the school, an African American named Michael, to succeed him as president of the Black Student Union.

***

The investigation concluded in May, just before graduation. Warren decided not to walk the stage just as in high school. He was due to speak at the event but relinquished this opportunity to his presidential secretary, Gracie. Warren didn't even go to his accepted transfer achievement event. He took his transfer achievement certificate and then packed his office into a box. He thanked everyone, swore in the next student body president, who was an elderly woman from the History club, and never returned to the office.

In July of that summer in 2019, Warren was sent the results of the investigation. He read a lengthy transcript and summary of everything that was said in the interviews and who said it. Warren was thrilled because it had confirmed a lot of what he had felt and suspected, reaffirmed a lot of what he had been told, and was glad to finally get his truth out in print. He reached the bottom of the results and saw that he had been absolved of any wrongdoing and that no evidence of harassment was found. He was innocent of his enemies' claims and overcame their schemes. However, as Warren continued to read, he saw that they also found him to be more than likely to retaliate and very likely to intimidate. Warren found this astonishing as well as amusing. First, it made him realize that maybe he didn't handle everything so well up to that point, but he was glad he did something. Secondly, he knew the main reason the investigator and human resources even bothered to add that detail after saying he was innocent was due to a meeting Warren had with the director of human resources while he was still president. In the meeting, he discussed his concerns with them hiring a student services coordinator who was friends with Pablo. The director dismissed his concerns as being temporary and not enough to disqualify the candidate. When Warren explained that another candidate, who happened to be the other clerk opposite Pablo in his office, was removed from the final stage wrongfully, she dismissed that, too, as the clerk having had too much history within the organization. Warren agreed, and to be honest, he really did not care if the clerk got it. In fact, he didn't want him to. He just wanted to gauge how he would dethrone the student services coordinator from her newly-hired position. He felt her conflict of interest with Pablo had run its course and was bothered that it ran interference on him in the middle of his last semester at the school and as president. Warren wanted her to go, but the director of human resources dismissed Warren's complaints as a conflict with his former position on the hiring committee and he left her office.

Warren, who knew the clerk had a big mouth and had a tendency of rushing to take credit for work before its originator or performer could text him and told him that the only reason he didn't make it to the final round of the hiring process, despite that he qualified and was in the top three of candidates the last time Warren checked, was because the new-hire was friends with people in human resources and in administration. The clerk then ran over to the administration building and into human resources and raised hell.

The next day, Warren got an invitation to a meeting with the director of human resources again. He already knew that he was in trouble. When he sat in the chair opposite the director's desk, he braced for her wrath and she let him have it. Red in the face and hot in temperament, she told Warren he would never serve on another human resource or hiring committee, that he should have recused himself from the hiring process if he had reservations about any of the candidates, and how he ultimately ruined a task that was done and now had to possibly be done over. She told him the position would have to return to the talent pool, and a possible recast and rehire may have to take place. Warren sat in silence for a moment, watching as the director calmed and meditated on her fury. He knew she had prior military experience and he felt she delivered a military-ass-chowing. Telling her what she wanted to hear, he said he regretted ruining her process and that he was prepared not to serve on another one of her hiring committees. He said he would learn from the mistake and she dismissed him without another word.

After graduation, Warren decided on Fresno Pacific University and successfully transferred. When he got the investigation results and saw what Pablo had said of him, he didn't hesitate or wait to text him everything he thought of him in return. Warren called him out for doing most of the stuff he had accused him of doing and things that Warren had even voiced concerns to him about. He also called him jealous, told him to avoid him in life, and reminded him that his greatest achievement as student body president of Merced College came when he had him kicked out of the office. Warren then circulated the messages throughout Pablo's friendship circle until Warren got a call from a friendly police officer who left a brief, kind voice message on his phone asking if he needed to talk. Warren took the hint that left Pablo alone. In September, the girl who accused him of harassment, sent a lengthy text message that said she was sorry for engaging in petty behavior and apologized for her actions. He accepted her apology and didn't respond when she sent another. Warren was at peace. He had won.

Chapter XIII: 2020

After Warren graduated from Merced College in May of 2019, he had a voice message from Dominic telling him he was back in Vallejo. Then he got a call from Aunt Sheryl confirming what Dominic had told him. She said he relapsed and began doing drugs again and that his behavior had grown out of control. Warren's Uncle Al had been in Las Vegas at the time visiting and paid for his ticket to get on a greyhound. This was interesting to him because he had also bought Warren's greyhound ticket when he sent him to Stockton fourteen years prior. When Warren tried to call Dominic back, he got his voicemail. When he tried again a week later, it was disconnected.

This was around the time Warren received his Ancestry DNA results and, for the first time, became fascinated with his being, although it only confirmed much of what he already knew. He also built a family tree. Then, over the summer, Warren applied for employment with Merced County Behavioral Health and Recovery Services. He had been working as an embedded peer mentor at school and at the front desk of a hotel earlier in the year, but he needed something that aligned better with his new and updated goals.

Willow had also been working for Merced County since they moved there in 2017. She had transferred to Behavioral

Health and became a mental health worker and highly encouraged Warren to apply, telling him his childhood background would give him the life- experience needed to become a peer support specialist. In August, he was hired. The couple sold their 2005 Ford Focus that had reached 355,000 miles and bought a 2013 Ford Fusion. Then, having taken half of the Fall semester off to recover from the year's stress, Warren did his onboarding training and then started his job as a peer support specialist at the county. Warren loved his job. Willow was stationed across the street at an old youth campus and he was stationed at the Adult Wellness Center in the main building, which was newly remodeled and refurbished after being funded by the Mental Health Services Act. It used to be the town's old hospital, the one most of the locals were born in until they built the new Mercy Hospital in North Merced. It was abandoned until the county and state needed a new mental health services hub in the area. Warren's job was to socialize with consumers who suffered from severe mental health, personality, and behavioral disorders such as schizophrenia, bipolar, anxiety, and depression. He was put in charge of the men's group and spent each day of work getting to know the stories of those around him to better understand them. He discovered that listening, being nonjudgmental and understanding, were the top three ingredients to a successful healing and recovery process. Occasionally, he'd have to deal with an unruly or disgruntled consumer, but at the end of every day, he knew they were part of the same family. Warren realized that when he was around his consumers, his own anxieties, fears and even voices would settle. He felt he was where he was needed.

***

In January 2020, Warren began his first semester at Fresno Pacific University. He was an English major at Merced College, but when he transferred, he put in a request to switch studies to business administration. Warren had reflected on his work and leadership experience up to that point and felt he had much to learn. He felt how he handled issues in the past was aggressive, manipulative, and chaotic. Warren wanted to get better, so he vowed to do better. The school approved his change of study and he joined the rest of his business cohort on the first day of school. In his second week of the program, he was selected by his peers and got paid a stipend to be his cohort's class representative.

After completing the first two classes of the program, the world stopped as everyone was informed that a deadly virus known as COVID-19, or the Coronavirus, had escaped a lab facility or meat market in Wuhan, China and was spreading rapidly across the globe. On January 21st, the Center for Disease Control confirmed the first US Coronavirus case and on January 23rd, Wuhan fell under quarantine. The US declared a public health emergency on February 3rd and on March 13th, President Trump declared the novel virus a national emergency. Then, on March 19th, the day before Warren and Willow's one-year wedding anniversary, California became the first state to issue a statewide stay-at-home order. Also, radios, TV advertisements, and grocery store intercoms began broadcasting face-mask reminders, requirements, and laws. Warren didn't mind it, he had spent the last thirty years in his home and in his own head. He was comfortable and now the world got to share the experience with him. However, while most of the state had to file for unemployment benefits, he and Willow were deemed essential workers and were still required to arrive at work every day. They didn't complain and knew that they were servants of the public and therefore, had an obligation. Eventually, Willow's building closed and they regulated her to work remotely from home. Warren didn't get that luxury, he still arrived at the Adult Wellness Center in the big main building of Behavioral Health and Recovery Services every day.

The Wellness Center felt different to him. It wasn't bustling with consumers of all types and backgrounds anymore and no longer were doctors, nurses, and clinicians scrambling back and forth, ducking in and out of offices and cubicles to attend to them and their needs. The place was empty and quiet. There were times when Warren would sit in the middle of the center and wonder how it came to this. He had avoided such an institution his whole life and now he stood in one, all to himself. When his division purchased clothing and hygiene kits to donate to the homeless community before they got placed into hotel quarantine, Warren was on the front lines, bagging kits, folding clothes, and packing everything into boxes. He helped load out into county vehicles and would do shifts in the main lobby, screening patients for the virus. When he wasn't busy helping with outreach, he was on the phone calling consumers from his caseload and after outreach and operations slowed, he decided to do something more productive with his time. Warren had always wanted to tell his story and encouraged others in his family to do the same. At work, he learned that another good way to heal from one's history was to put it into a narrative and tell it as a story. The process had confirmed much of what he had known to be true. He knew he had made the right choice. When the consumers returned, Warren thought he would have something to give them and this story, he felt, was his gift.

**

On May 25th, 2020, an African American man named George Floyd Jr. was killed during an arrest after he tried to pass a counterfeit $20 bill. A white police officer had knelt on his neck for more than eight minutes. Then, beginning on May 26th and continuing even to this day, protests and civil unrest erupted across the United States and internationally. While the majority of the protests were peaceful, demonstrations in some cities escalated into riots, looting, and street skirmishes with police. CBS News compiled a list of 164 black men and women who were killed by the police from January 1st to August 31st. Cries to defund the police began to spread across the nation. When protests were organized for Merced, Warren felt it was his duty and obligation to participate. He had been president of the Black Student Union, Student Body President, and now worked for the county. His entire being told him to march. So, when London, a buddy of his who he met when he volunteered at the food bank, called him and asked if he wanted to go, Warren said yes.

Warren marched with London up and down Olive Avenue in Merced with a crowd numbering into the hundreds. Cars honked and people chanted in support while others, with big American trucks and big waving American flags, posted across the street from the meeting area and even patrolled up and down the street as they marched to intimidate and flex their own views. One truck pulled up next to Warren with their flag and he complimented them on it. He said it was his flag too.

Epilogue

After graduating and achieving honors from Fresno Pacific University in 2021, Warren got accepted into Arizona State University to study for a master's degree in organizational leadership. This was around the time he got moved to the medical services division at work to support a telehealth psychiatrist with consumers and appointments. One of the reasons Warren chose Arizona State University was because Dominic and his family were from the state. He felt this was his chance to rise above the family once and for all. Halfway through his first and only year in the master's program, Warren was accepted into Arizona State's doctor of behavioral health program at the College of Health Solutions with an emphasis in management. The psychiatrist he had been assigned to at work, Dr. Ly, wrote him a good letter of recommendation.

With the benefits from his county job, Warren got many health issues that have plagued him since adolescence checked and remedied. He also saw a therapist and vented out all the years of pain, trials, and tribulations he experienced. In doing so, he felt liberated. There were times he felt wounds were cut back open, but he felt it necessary for the healing process. He even began to have nightmares of events that took place during his childhood. He stuck with his counselor anyway, Mr. Hubbell, and eventually graduated from therapy around the time he graduated with his master's degree. To give back to his community and to serve those who were very much like him and who still need help in their path to wellness and recovery, Warren filed articles of incorporation and founded a nonprofit company with several others on May 28, 2022. The purpose and mission of the company is to provide residential mental health and substance use disorder housing. Through Warren's studies and employment, he discovered a vicious cycle in that those with mental illnesses were more prone to health and societal problems, including homelessness and violence, if there weren't community support and housing options in place to help them. He saw a never-ending cycle of crime spikes, family destruction, and community disruption regarding those who refused to get help for their mental illness or substance use disorders. Dominic ended back up homeless and on meth after Warren's wedding and he didn't bother to find him again because he understands more than most that his dad will never seek help until he is ready to get help. Warren remembered a time when Dominic seemed normal. Things changed when Dominic lost his job, became homeless, and his girlfriend left him. He fell back onto old habits he had before he went to jail for thirteen-plus years. Warren, in his new dream and career choice, decided to help those like his dad who didn't have much help growing up and coming out of jail, hospital, or a crisis. With the residential facilities Warren's company plans to build and operate, he hopes homelessness can be reduced, care can be properly provided to those who need it, and people can be integrated back into their communities and families so they may contribute to society, participate in family affairs, and be a decent human being and citizen.

Afterword

In reflection, Warren saw everything that happened in his life happened for a reason. He realized God was with him each day of his life. Although he struggled and endured difficult obstacles and people, he knew God never let him go and helped him overcome them. He was always there, fighting for him at work, in school, and in love.

Warren forgave his family. He felt he couldn't move forward in life or live peacefully and with happiness if he didn't. He reached out to Rhonda, engaged her in forgiveness, and then she shared with him their family history and any other questions he had about the family, its history, and life. When he told her about the problems he had at college, she shared with him a story of her own that was very much similar. During the last four years of her life, she made a strong and sincere attempt to repair her relationship with Warren and inspired him to finish school, love his wife, and do the right thing. She also hoped he wouldn't keep too many bad memories of her after she leaves earth. He truly forgave her. In the month of September, in the year 2022, Rhonda succumbed to her health issues and passed away. Warren wept. He prayed for Christ to receive and keep her. One thing Warren realized when he was angry at his family for so many years was that if he stood mad at them long enough, then he surely would become just like them, and if he had not gone through what he did in life, he never would've become the person he is today. Warren wanted to be free, so he forgave everyone. He started with Paul, his mother's tormentor, then Christian, Uncle Al, Uncle Victor, Dominic, and Grandma Peace, and worked his way all the way up to the present. He was even able to finally connect with Uncle Curt's son and apologize for what happened twelve years prior. They have grown close ever since. When he had completed his forgiveness streak, he realized he didn't do it so much for himself but mainly for the glory of God and to chase after His heart.

It is with sincere hope this book can be used as a light and a guide, after the Bible, to help you overcome your own obstacles. Whatever it is you, a relative or a friend are going through. We encourage you to remain hopeful, guard your heart, and be resilient.

You will live.

CPSIA information can be obtained
at www.ICGtesting.com
Printed in the USA
BVHW052035261222
654951BV00015B/653